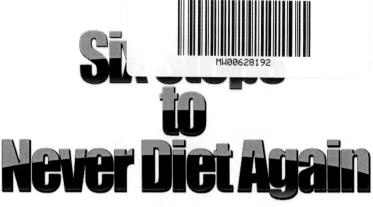

Six Steps to Never Diet Again

Free Yourself from the Diet Trap

Myrna Haag

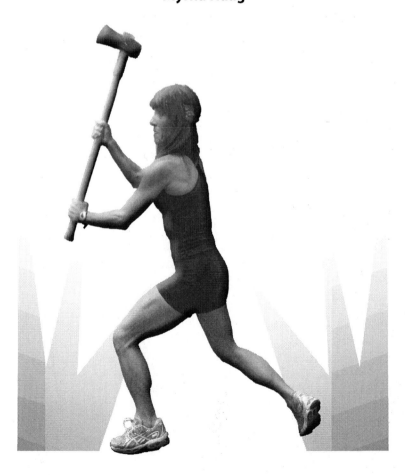

Myrna Haag offers programs materials and coaching to help people improve their lifestyle.
Contact: www.myrnahaag.com   813-253-3999 ext 201

Copyright © 2009 by Myrna Haag,
Library of Congress Cataloging-in-Publication Data

ISBN # 978-0-9824938-0-9

Published by Myrna Publishing,
A division of Myrna LLC,
1700 S. MacDill Ave. Suite #260,
Tampa, Fl. 33629

Printed in the United States of America

Interior layout and book cover design; by Myrna Haag with the help of Whitney Lasseter and cover photography by Tom Couture.

Editors: Bonnie Hearn and Beverly Mallassi
Printer: digital press, Tampa Fl.
Permission credits:
Quote by Dr. Amen from Making a Good Brain Great
References from: www.mypyramid.gov
www.American Heart association

This book is dedicated to my mom and dad,
Adeline and Manuel Garcia,
Through their wisdom and love all things are possible.

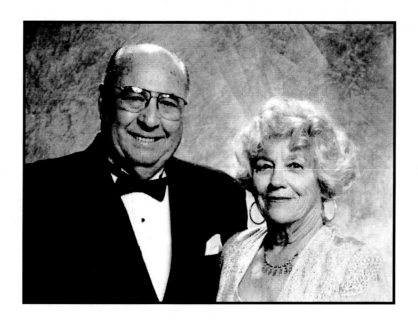

Acknowledgments

Special thanks goes to all friends and family for supporting and encouraging me through this process.

To my mom and dad for always being there for me.

To my family, Gary, Samantha and Gavin for having the patience, and love to see me through.

To Dr. Karen Mutter and Lynne Walder for sharing your knowledge and seeing the potential in the six steps.

To Don Ardell for your intellectual sweep.

To Beverly Melasi Haag for encouraging me to finish the dog-gone book, and then doing a final edit.

To Angela Ohler for sharing your super brilliance to help me see how it should be and can be.

To Catie Whelan Rood for constantly reminding me that God is holding my hand.

To Bonnie Hearn for editing and giving me the last burst of confidence .

To Denise McClellan for telling me it was good.

To Natalie Ritenour and Whitney Lasseter for believing in the process and using it to help others.

To Angie Arnst for volunteering your time to help me host clinics for our community.

To Barb Couture for having that sixth sense and using it to encourage me.

Contents

Forward

Myrna's Six Steps to Living Healthy

Many diseases in humans are directly or indirectly caused by malnutrition, a general term for a medical condition caused by improper or inadequate diet and nutrition. When we think of malnutrition, we think of very thin people in countries far away. But malnutrition can result in both underweight or overweight conditions. And in this country, we have far more overweight than underweight individuals.

Obesity, a serious form of malnutrition, is rapidly becoming an epidemic in America due to the availability and low cost of fast foods and packaged foods. These foods can also be highly addictive because of the imbalance they create in the body. Another explanation of our rapidly growing overweight population may be our general disconnect from the concept of food as nourishment. We have gotten farther and farther away from the source of the foods that we eat and we have lost the connection between the foods we eat and how they make us feel every day.

If ever there was a time when a clear and practical guide was essential to help people learn how to gain better health through the proper use of food....it is NOW! Almost two-thirds (about 66%) of U.S. adults age 20 or older are overweight -- about 62% of women and around 71% of men. The prevalence of being overweight has steadily increased over the years among both genders, all ages, racial and ethnic groups and educational levels. Why is this important? Because it is clear from medical research that Americans who are obese/ overweight are more likely to suffer from many chronic diseases, such as heart disease (including stroke and hypertension), diabetes, and cancers of the uterus, breast, prostate, colon and rectum. Obesity is also linked to high cholesterol, gallstones and gallbladder disease, gout and osteoarthritis, complications of pregnancy, poor female reproductive health (such as menstrual irregularities, infertility, irregular ovulation), bladder control problems (such as stress incontinence) and psychological disorders (such as depression, eating disorders, distorted body image and low self- esteem).

Obesity-related illness results in hundreds of thousands of preventable deaths each year in the United States and billions of dollars in health care costs.

In this era of cheap, fast food, it is not only the overweight and obese who are experiencing health problems; even normal weight individuals living on a highly processed, high fat and sugar diet are seeking help for chronic fatigue, depression, fibromyalgia and any number of inflammatory and auto-immune diseases. Many of these people are given medications to combat their symptoms which continue to fuel a sea of imbalanced hormones and neurochemicals that keep them feeling chronically unwell.

An equally great tragedy is that mainstream medicine is ill-equipped to handle these problems. Yes, there are medications available to treat the many symptoms and diseases that result from improper nutrition, but this is downstream medicine—treating the symptoms rather than addressing the cause of the problem. This is like spending all of our money and resources on cleaning up the floods rather than fixing the dam. Many doctors will ask their patients to lose weight, but few are adequately trained to teach them how to do so.

Very little time is devoted in medical school to the study of nutrition. The truth is that the chemicals in our foods effect how our body systems function. Food has the power to wreak havoc on our system and also to balance it as well. We must begin to think about food in a different way-- food can be the very medicine to help us heal! Simply eating the right balance of foods and eliminating the foods that are toxic to our system is an extremely effective and powerful medicine in its own right.

It is in this concept that Myrna has created this very excellent and useful guide to anyone who is struggling with health concerns and weight issues. Through 30 years of working with clients as a certified fitness trainer and through her own personal experience of becoming a nationally ranked triathlete in her late 40s, Myrna has spent most of her life studying and helping people find their way to a healthier life. Myrna will be the first to tell you, "this is not a diet book!" And thank goodness for that because a search for diet books on Amazon.com reveals over 21,500 in print!

What makes this book different is that it is not about the kinds of foods you can and cannot have. It's not about deprivation or miracle cures. It is about empowering people with basic tools to understand how to use food to feed and nourish the body in a way that creates biochemical balance. These tools are presented in a logical, easy to follow 6 step process that is effective, scientifically sound and transcends financial status.

It is a program that has been developed and refined over the past 15 years and can be followed whether you are on food stamps or own your own grocery store. It works because, when you fuel the body with the proper balance of proteins, carbohydrates, fats, and water, the cravings and cycle of biochemical imbalance can be interrupted. These are 6 basic principles that can change your life and permanently improve your health.

Part of what makes Myrna and this 6 step process so remarkable is her work with the indigent and underprivileged population. For over 20 years Myrna has worked with women in homeless shelters through the Salvation Army and YMCA programs. She has been a passionate and tireless advocate for this often neglected part of our society that, ironically, are often the most overweight.

This has been the proving ground for the success of this 6 step program. Here, in the most difficult of circumstances, she has empowered thousands of people to restore balance and thus decrease physical symptoms associated with malnutrition, improve self-esteem through education and exercise, and ultimately reduce their body weight by utilizing the 6 steps program. I cannot say enough about Myrna's inspirational service to our community in this way.

We are in a time of serious issues related to healthcare funding and availability. Often, the general public feels powerless waiting for the government to change the system. However, we do have the power to take responsibility for our own health. How do we do this? First and foremost through the foods we choose to put in our bodies.

Of course there are many factors that influence our health, some not in our control. But what we choose to eat every day is something we can do to make a positive impact on our health and quality of life. In this way, each one of us can be a part of the solution to our healthcare crisis by decreasing the burden of healthcare costs. This book is an invaluable guide to making these educated choices about your own self care.

So make a choice for a balanced body **today.** Read on to learn about these 6 steps so that you can start to enjoy more energy, weight regulation, and personal empowerment that comes with taking care of yourself. Whether you are an elite athlete, an over-weight mom, or someone who simply wishes to improve their health and develop an efficient and balanced body, these 6 Steps will serve you well.

Karen L. Mutter, D.O.
Board Certified Internal Medicine
Board Certified Holistic Medicine

"Everyone has a doctor in him or her; we just have to help it in its work. The natural healing force within each one of us is the greatest force in getting well. Our food should be our medicine. Our medicine should be our food."

Hippocrates, Greek Physician (460 BC–370 BC)

Preface

Almost thirty years ago I had a doctor tell me I had a predisposition to be over weight. I took after my father's side of the family, and as long as I didn't gain 20-30 pounds I would be fine. The doctor gave me a clean bill of health and told me I will need to watch my weight the rest of my life, especially since there is a family history of diabetes. He recommended a diet of fruits vegetables and lean meats. For someone who just turned twenty, it seemed unfair. The thought of being on a diet my whole life was really depressing.

I suppose all the years of swimming in high school just covered up my overweight tendencies, and some serious eating issues. It is difficult to explain to someone how a hot fudge sundae or a soft warm chewy chocolate chip cookie can be your best friend one minute, and then destroy your life the next. I knew the real challenge would be to try and not gain 100 pounds over the next 20 years. I could live with an extra 15-20 pounds, but 100 pounds would limit everything I do. I knew the doctor was right, no matter how hard I tried to loose weight, I would eventually gain it back, as if being fat was the body I was suppose to have; it was my genetic fate.

That was then …this is now!

For the last thirty years I have studied the truth and applied the methods that it takes to live lean and healthy permanently. Trying to live lean and healthy in America is an impossible challenge. It has nothing to do with dieting, long hours of exercise, or some genetic code, it has everything to do with a process you can control. The six steps explained in this book are the beginning of that process. It has worked for me and the thousands of people I have helped and it will work for you too.

The information in this book is really powerful and you need to read it. I know this message won't reach everyone, but for those willing to learn, it has, and continues to change lives. It has nothing to do with food, and has everything to do with you around food. It is a chemical process, It is a state you put your body in, most the time, unintentionally. It is about understanding how to keep your body balanced through the foods you eat. If you're balanced, food cravings go away, you aren't a victim of food and the hold it has on you. It is not about portion control through deprivation. It is about keeping your body in a chemical place, naturally, where you live lean and healthy because your body puts you there.

The world tells us being over weight is our fault...we don't exercise enough... we are lazy and lack self control. Wrong!! It is not ...and we are not!

About the Author

Myrna Haag lives in Tampa Florida, has been married 23 years and has two children.

Myrna Haag provides healthy lifestyle coaching for individuals and organizations who demonstrate a strong desire to be healthy and are committed to achieving success in healthy lifestyle behaviors. Myrna's goal is to empower people to live a healthy lifestyle using simple strategies that anyone can apply to their life, resulting in significant improvements in their quality of life.

Myrna Haag has worked and volunteered in the fitness industry for over 25 years, empowering homeless and disadvantaged communities to live balanced healthy lives. She is a competitive tri-athlete. She was ranked fourth in the 2004 United States Triathlon Age Group (45-50) National Championships and eleventh in the United States Triathlon Age Group World Championships. She serves as a personal and group exercise trainer, who has helped thousands of individuals achieve their goals of a healthier lifestyle, through her athletic accomplishments, and by working with others to achieve their goals. She has studied which nutrition and exercise methods work and which do not.

Through lectures, workshops, cooking and fitness demonstrations, as well as participation in community-based organizations Myrna has spread her six step healthy lifestyle message to thousands of people.

You can contact Myrna at **www.myrnahaag.com**.

INTRODUCTION

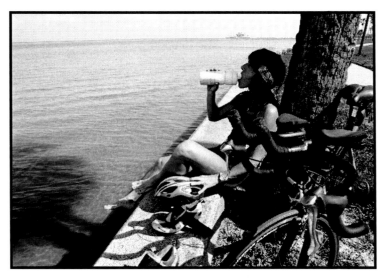

Myrna relaxing after an afternoon workout

What Feels Good

When I began coaching weight-loss groups, I never anticipated that having a lot of energy would be something these groups feared or had to be convinced was a better way to live. Stupid me. I thought I was being motivating as I explained all the new energy they would have, how the world would feel and seem different, how they would feel more alive and blissful, and have a beautiful lean body to show for it. The more I talked, the more stressed out they became. Just listening to me made them feel as if it was something they could never have; it would require changing too much, something they weren't able to do.

Especially in groups that had a lot of weight to lose. Their being overweight allowed them to escape from the world. Comfort foods created a fogged feeling that calmed and relaxed them; a numbing feeling of indifference. It was not exciting, but it was very safe, and being safe is what these seriously overweight people felt they needed most. Their obese lifestyle was a way of protecting themselves, and nothing felt better than feeling safe.

Those who have lost over 100 pounds and have kept it off living a healthy lifestyle have told me that before this energetic, blissful life became something they wanted more than the safe, drugged-numb feeling, they had to first learn to love themselves. They had to come to a place where they felt they were worth it. It had to be more about loving the body they had, no matter how overweight it had become, and how much they blamed it for all their un-happiness. They had to empower themselves before they could get to the point where what I said made any sense. Although empowerment is my last step in this book, in working with this group of dangerously obese people, I realized it needed to be first.

Empowerment is when you connect with yourself. Without empowerment, you cannot succeed at being or staying healthy. In fact, you are pretty much stuck in every aspect of your life. It's hard to decide what is more important: to dive right into the food aspect of the six steps, or work on the empowerment step first.

I understand where you're at, and this book will show you how to fix it. The real question is: are you ready to accept it? You have to empower yourself to be ready before you can really make these six steps work. Even if you're not ready now, I still believe having the information can and will make a difference for when you are.

"If you are ready, this book will change your life!"

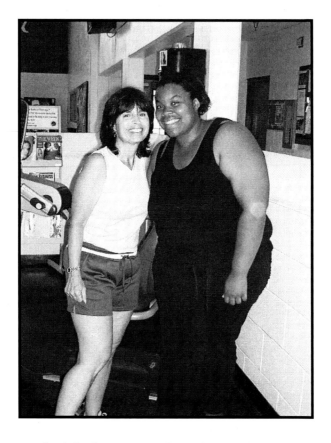

Natalie (left), lost 70 pounds on the six step program. She now coaches others to live balanced.

One

Why You Feel Trapped

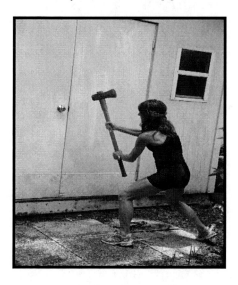

Myrna breaks from food addiction.

What if This is Your Reality?

Ever feel as if your body holds you back? Are you fatigued or depressed? Does your normal routine seem overwhelming at times? Do you gain weight easily and struggle to lose even two to three pounds? Does it seem as if you're trapped into making bad food choices? Do so-called *comfort foods* call out to you as a reward after a stressful day? Does your whole body seem to run in slow motion? Are you afraid to exert yourself because you fear injury or just plain lack motivation?

If you answered "yes" to any or all of these questions, you're just like millions of other people who struggle with energy level, weight gain, and overall fatigue; people who separate their physical selves from their mental, emotional and spiritual selves. People who create a protective shield while trying to restore self-worth. Separating yourself emotionally and physically becomes a necessary process when you have tried everything else, and you feel that there is no way out.

Do you feel as if when the world looks at you, it passes judgment on your physical self and doesn't see the real you?

You Can't Separate Your Body From Who You Are

Are there times you wish you could separate the real you from the flesh you're trapped in? The hard reality is, this fleshy cage limits what you can do, and how much you are able to enjoy your life. You know in your heart this overweight, flabby, fatigued person isn't who you really are. No matter how hard you try, you seem to come back to this depressing place, as if it is the physical body you are destined to have, and you have learned to accept it.

What if You Want to be Lean and Healthy, But You Feel Trapped?

Being overweight and tired all the time feels as if you are in a prison you can never escape. Even if you want to change to a healthier lifestyle, there are just too many challenges to overcome. You tell yourself that you simply do not have the motivation or time to take on one more energy-draining battle. Not even if it gives you energy? The problem is that it takes energy to get there. Perhaps you are convinced that it takes too much energy, time, money, and personal commitment, and that it is a luxury you just can't afford.

A Quick Diet Seems Like The Solution

As soon as you get to that low point, you begin a diet that promises a *new you* in 30 days. How many times have you announced your goal of losing weight to the world, then ventured off with your lettuce leaves and low-fat dressing, surrounded by food you wished you could have but knew you couldn't? You may lose weight in 30 days on some quick torture-like program, but are you really solving the problem? Do you know for sure you won't gain it back? Are you really going to be able to give up your favorite foods?

Most Quick Fixes are Temporary Fixes

Nothing works permanently until you change inside; the way you think about food, and the way you think about yourself around food. What we are really talking about here is making the right choices because you want to, not because you have to.

Most people can't imagine they could change how they think about food. It is hard to believe you can rewire your brain to not crave your favorite comfort foods. After all, you love the taste and short-term pleasure of eating your favorite foods. Is it really possible to stop the urge to want more, even when the voice inside your head is telling you to take more? The reason is because you haven't worked on **you**! Your inside stuff. Yes, that's right. Everything you have tried has been external, and simply doesn't work.

Losing weight and keeping it off *permanently* has little to do with dieting or excessive exercise programs. It is not about external influences. There is no magic formula, diet or equipment that is going to make this happen, because it isn't about external influences. It has everything to do with you and how you are wired internally.

You Can Rewire Yourself!

The abuse stops when you make good choices, because doing so makes you feel good, not because it is something you have to do. Is it possible to crave a workout or really want a big bowl of vegetables instead of a decadent piece of cake? What if French fries, chips, or some other salty, crispy, sweet, or creamy something that has been your true downfall was no longer a comfort food for you? In fact, what if you were indifferent to foods that in the past were hard to stay away from?

Imagine your exercise program being something you really looked forward to! The real goal is to have the program that keeps you healthy and lean be the one you love doing, where you don't think about what you *should* or shouldn't eat. Contrary to what the people who want to take your money (*and* your life) will tell you, you really can't take a lifetime of bad habits and expect a new you in six weeks. Sometimes it can take six weeks just to rewire your brain.

The Ultimate Goal is to Change How You Feel About Food

You cannot remove food from your life. Thus, you have to change how you feel around food. That is the only way you will ever be free, living a lean, healthy life you enjoy, and having the body to prove it.

No longer being a victim of food means you get to choose what you eat; something you alone design, with foods you truly enjoy. It has to work for you, not someone else. Keep in mind that naturally thin people don't follow a diet plan. They are free to eat what they want. You also will need to have free choice. Otherwise, it will never work.

Reprogramming is all about a process – not a program or special diet. You have to be taught how to play the game and learn the rules for success. It is not about special foods that make you thin, forbidden foods you sneak when no one is looking, or the long hours of exercise that are boring and feel like torture. Living a healthy, lean lifestyle is about living a life you love that loves you back. The love is reflected in the energetic, lean healthy body you carry around.

Are Naturally Thin People Wired Differently?

I'm sure you have met naturally thin people who tell you they can eat anything, and as much as they desire. Have you ever really spent the day or several days with them, and watched what and how they eat? They may order a rich meal with loads of calories, eat half or maybe only a quarter of the food, and be done. They order dessert and eat three bites. They are the ones who have candy sitting on their desk at work, and the candy bowl is always full. Most people could never have a bowl of candy sitting on their desks in fear that they would consume the whole bowl the moment no one was looking.

What makes these people different is that there is no internal battle. They desire only half of a decadent meal, and eat three bites of a dessert and feel 100 percent satisfied. Others could feel deprived by only eating three bites of dessert, or wouldn't be able to stop themselves from overeating, because that's what feels right to them.

To someone who struggles with weight, leaving half a meal creates an internal voice that tells them they are depriving themselves of the entire meal. A naturally thin person eats half the meal and feels satisfied. The difference is that the thin person has no internal battle. Even when half the meal remains on their plate, they are eating whatever they want as much as they want.

The key to permanent weight loss is to get you in that mind set, too, but unlike some naturally thin people, you will be more empowered because you will know how it works and how to stay there.

If You Are Overweight You Are Not Healthy

Maybe you believe that being overweight has no correlation to your health. Perhaps you believe you can follow a drastic weight-loss program (or surgery), and once you lose all of that weight, then you will work on being healthy. Wrong!

People believe once they lose weight, they will be free of a lifetime of bad habits and suddenly live this healthy life. Once the weight is gone, they will miraculously be motivated to exercise and always choose the right foods, and never again be tempted.

> *Permanent weight loss means your health must come first. Otherwise your body will never allow you to keep the weight off.*

Wrong! Less than 2% actually keep the weight off mainly because the only focus is weight loss. They don't understand it isn't about losing weight. It is really about keeping it off, and that means you have to be healthy.

Unfortunately, people get trapped in the quick-fix weight loss programs, diet aids and low-calorie/no-carbohydrate diet programs that are only a temporary approach that will pack on the pounds even faster than before.

Being Overweight and Believing You Are Healthy is Called Denial

Most people believe as long as they haven't been diagnosed with a serious illness they are healthy. Many have experienced a positive diagnosis from their doctors, and yet some suffer from symptoms of fatigue, depression, lack of motivation, and all-over aches and pains.

Normal blood work from your doctor means that you aren't suffering from a detectable disease *yet,* and that's about it. If you're dealing with the fatigue, the depression, and all of those aches and pains, you're not living a high quality of life. Meanwhile, the patient sits in the doctor's office carrying 30-50 pounds of excess fat, getting a *temporary* clean bill of health. Of course, the doctor himself may also carry an additional 30-50 pounds of fat. Both are in denial, because being overweight means something is missing. Let's face it, most people who are obese, don't want to be obese, and know what foods make them overweight and which ones don't.

If you believe you're overweight because of a challenging past, you are finding an excuse. It doesn't help, and it isn't the real problem. There are plenty of naturally thin people who have a murky past and a stressful life, but don't need food to relieve them or make them forget. Sure, food can be a comforting drug, but it doesn't have to be. Your body is telling your brain it needs it.

This is usually all because of some imbalance you have unintentionally created. These imbalances not only make you eat foods you really don't want, they also lead to poor health.

Living Healthy Requires Balance

Living healthy means you know how to create harmony and balance, which comes down to the truth: If you are seriously overweight, you are not healthy. Focusing only on weight loss means you may lose the weight, but you won't keep it off. Why? Because you have missed the big picture entirely. In short, you are overweight because you don't understand how to be healthy. It is all about how to keep your body balanced.

> The only way you can rewire your brain is to maintain balance in your body first. Otherwise, your body will control your brain.

Most people don't understand that the human body is a big bag of chemicals, and unless you know how to balance these chemicals, you will struggle with your weight your entire life, which ultimately leads to poor health. If you try and lose weight without understanding how to maintain balance then you actually set yourself up to be fatter.

Being lean has everything to do with being healthy, but unless you know how to get there correctly you will **not** have a permanent solution. In other words, your brain and body will be in battle forever, and you will have an overweight body to prove it.

Stop Believing That a Thin Person is a Healthy Person

Keep in mind, just because someone is thin, either naturally, or because they work at it, doesn't mean they know how to maintain balance and have a healthy body to back it. Just because they are living a lifestyle that allows them to have a low body weight, doesn't mean they are healthy and full of energy. You can still be thin and not be healthy. There are thin people who believe success is a number on the scale. Every morning is a ritual with the bathroom scales that dictates their food intake for the rest of the day.

They're still victims, still following a deprived lifestyle of all the foods they can't eat. In a word, *yo-yo*. In two words— *trapped and struggling*. Being thin doesn't mean a *dog gone* thing! It just means they are thin.

> *Permanent weight loss has everything to do with how healthy you are. How healthy you are has everything to do with knowing how to keep your body balanced.*

The truth is, some weight loss programs are very unhealthy! Bottom line, if you lose weight in an unhealthy manner, you have only lost weight, which means it isn't permanent, because you haven't changed your lifestyle. It will all come back! Losing weight is not the answer, and to just focus on weight loss will lead to failure, believe me. The best method is when weight loss becomes, not the *focus*, but the *result* of a healthy lifestyle.

Know why? Unless you figure out how to keep your body balanced, permanent weight loss will be a struggle. Just because you are losing weight doesn't mean you are balanced or that you are healthy. In fact, weight loss without regard to health is a disaster! It can create an imbalance that makes you worse off than before your weight-loss attempt.

The Rewiring Process in Myrna's Six Steps Keeps Balance

This book will teach you a process, not a diet. It has worked for thousands of people just like you, people who didn't think it was possible to change how they felt around food. After all, there's little chance our food environment will change. Unless you figure out how to change how you feel around food, you'll always be a victim of food. The only way a lean, healthy body is permanent is when it becomes a lifestyle, not a diet. Those naturally thin people we talked about don't have abusive internal battles going on in their brains. The only way the rewiring process can begin to take place is when your body is balanced, and not causing an internal battle with your brain.

The six-step process will teach you how to keep your body balanced, with foods you enjoy. It is a building process, and as you slowly change the way you think, you'll find your food choices will also change. You'll be surprised with the foods you'll eventually grow to love and crave the way you used to crave pizza and hot fudge sundaes. As your body becomes more balanced, you'll find you want healthier foods. No denial. No cravings. It's a natural progression. As your body becomes more balanced, it will naturally start to regulate itself. You'll be able to eat half a slice of pizza, or a few bites of dessert and feel 100% satisfied. In fact, when you are balanced you may find you don't want these foods at all. Once the cravings are gone, your brain will be able to think clearly.

What is Balance and How Does it Work?

Balance is the process of getting your body back to a neutral place; a state in which it is being properly nourished, protected from harmful substances, and ready to grow in strength and endurance. When everything is balanced, your body is able to tap into its natural regulatory system, which will eventually improve your health.

Poor health is usually a result of some regulatory problem. Your body is very smart, but your environment can be misleading it. It is difficult to have a smart body without smart foods. Additionally, you have to be smart about when you eat that food. Here's the deal. When you're on the typical fad diet, you aren't really making use of your body's natural regulatory system. You're keeping yourself from eating something you naturally want to eat. Bottom line: You are still imbalanced, and you maintain the weight loss by sheer force of will.

You know the drill. Eventually, you'll break down and go back to where you started. What you need to do is leverage your body's wisdom by putting yourself in balance and allowing your natural regulatory systems to kick in.

Look at your food environment—what is available for you to eat? If you are simply picking and choosing among bad foods, then your regulatory systems don't have a chance. Most likely, you don't even know that you're imbalanced. It probably seems almost normal to be overweight, tired, and depressed. Diets don't work because you haven't really worked on the problem. Diets just get the weight off. You eventually gain the weight back, and you are miserable in the process. It's hard to reprogram your brain when you feel hungry and deprived. When you're on a diet, it becomes all you think about. It becomes less about choice, and more about obedience.

Be Smart

Try to be as smart as your body is. Figure out how your body works, and work with it. When your body is balanced, there are no food binges, no sugar and fat addictions. Most of the problems with obesity have to do with the body trying to regulate an imbalance you unknowingly created. You have to learn how to balance the body, keeping all the regulatory systems running smoothly. The weight loss is really just the end result. The true benefit is the freedom and gain in energy.

Eating healthy food means you are eating foods that are rich in nutrients. Although this is better than not eating foods that have nutrients, it still doesn't mean you're eating the right combinations or amounts of what your body needs to regulate itself.

Eating Balanced Versus Eating Healthy

In my thirty years of helping others live lean, healthy lives, I have learned that if my clients don't understand how to keep their bodies balanced, they don't have the motivation to become educated on what food will provide the optimum health benefit. I have found that if you can work on helping people maintain their body weight with a process that empowers them to no longer be a victim of food, they eventually evolve to wanting – even craving – a higher quality of life that comes from eating healthy.

There is a difference between eating balanced and eating healthy. Eating food that is good for you doesn't mean you are balancing your body. It doesn't mean you are eating foods that keep your blood sugar level maintained, which regulates your hormones and ultimately affects your moods and energy level. It also doesn't mean you are eating foods that give you a faster metabolism, or that enable you to build more muscle tissue, which ultimately leads to a leaner body.

Eating healthy without understanding how to keep your body balanced can still be a disaster. You may be guarded against premature death, but your quality of life may be less than it could be. You could easily eat healthy and be 30 to 40 pounds overweight, because you'd still be a victim of food. On the other hand, you could be lean and maintain a chemical balance that would eventually kill you.

> *The point I'm trying to make is: You can still be overweight, tired and unmotivated to exercise eating organic food full of nutrients.*

Maybe you had a dinner containing enough antioxidants and vitamins for an elephant. Maybe your lunches consist of salad and fruit. Perhaps you buy only organic food, or eat only a vegetarian raw diet. Let me repeat. Although this food may be good for you, it doesn't mean you're eating food that will keep your body balanced, and that will allow you to tap into your natural source of energy.

The goal is to eat foods that keep you balanced, and supply your body exactly what it needs to prevent diseases. Unless you are balanced, it is really difficult to eat healthy.

Eating Healthy Food Doesn't Mean You are Balanced.

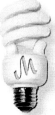

Being balanced is a chemical state you put your body in. Eating healthy is a conscious effort you make to find foods that have certain health benefits.

Look at your life, and decide.... Are you ready to learn how to keep balance with foods that are also good for you? If you say yes, then you'll want to know about the following six-step process.

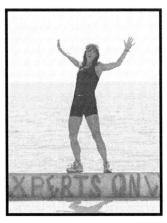

Myrna almost keeps balance

Wilting Rose story

Rose has a very small body frame. Clothes hang off her slender body. Despite the fact that she spends one to two hours per day exercising, she has little muscle to show for it. Rose's thinness is her badge of success. She is an advocate of juicing, believes in no animal food, and brags how she only eats organic raw vegetarian products. And what has that done for her, really? Well, Rose is surely protected from most cancers with a diet that is clean and rich in antioxidants.

Even though she is getting an abundance of vitamins and minerals, she complains every afternoon around 2 to 4 p.m. that she could use a nap. She is unable to exert herself and blames it on the fact that she just turned 45. The answer? Although Rose is eating foods that will bring her good health, she is not balancing her body correctly with her healthy food choices. Her diet consists of healthy food but she doesn't know how to balance these foods, which results in low energy which could lead to poor health. Balanced, healthy bodies are able to exert themselves, and Rose's can't. Balanced bodies grow muscles and gain high levels of strength and endurance. If Rose could learn how to balance her healthy food she would have an awesome body.

Just because you eat healthy food doesn't mean you will have a ton of energy. Muscular, lean, fit bodies only happen when there is energy driving the engines. Rose is unwilling to change. She believes feeling fatigued is a small price to pay for a perfect skinny figure. And if she's lucky, she will live a cancer-free, tired life! She's fearful that if she changes her formula of success she may gain weight, and she has accepted that more energy isn't part of her formula. There is little hope she will ever see the light. Her skinny lifestyle is supported by her peers, who place a higher value on looking good rather than feeling good. What neither they—nor Rose—has discovered is that nothing looks better than when you are balanced and full of energy..

TWO

HOW THE SIX-STEP PROCESS WORKS

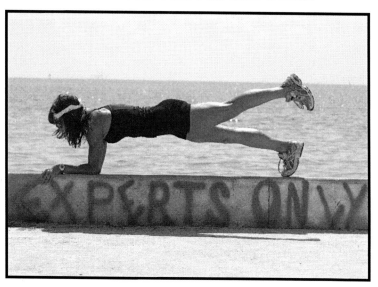

Myrna's seawall balancing act

A Process for Change

Most people don't start off on this journey towards a healthy life loving steamed broccoli and eager to work out. In fact, your six-step process may never include steamed broccoli, and you may never develop an interest in athletics. You have to start with a process that you can do at the place where you are now. As you begin the process of rewiring yourself, you will be amazed how you progress. You have to keep in mind that this is not another diet book. This is a book on learning a process for change. That is why you won't see menu plans and list of forbidden foods. You can't just turn to one section of this book and follow a diet. You have to un-derstand the concepts, the secrets that make it work, then decide what foods you choose to follow through within the six steps. Think of it this way: Living a healthy lifestyle is not a diet but a process. It has nothing to do with dieting and everything to do with the way you want to live.

The lifestyle you are about to learn centers around six steps. They may not make a lot of sense at first, but once you learn about the six-step process, you will be amazed how they will play a role in everything you eat. In order to have this process work for you, you have to commit yourself to go through each step and learn what makes each step special and what makes them magical when they are combined. To follow one or two steps is fabulous progress, but the real magic is when you do all six steps. That is when you will gain the greatest benefit. Even if you are not ready to start this program, you will get results just by having it in your brain, because you are not the first non-believer who ever walked away changed.

How Should I Read This Book to Learn the Process?

This book outlines six steps that will keep your body balanced. You can start with any step you want. If you normally read books back to front or skip around, whatever step you want to start with works fine. First, you have to be willing to educate yourself as to what makes the six-step process so special, and then you need to be willing to apply it to your life.

Because we are all so different, there will be some adjustments based on your own preferences. As you grow in the six-step process, your choices of foods may be very different than when you initially started. To be honest, everything you do may be different. What will remain the same is the process that got you there and keeps you there.

Here are the SIX STEPS that will balance the body and change your life when you follow them every day:

1. WATER
2. PROTEIN-FIBER COMBINATIONS
3. FATS
4. PORTIONS
5. MOVEMENT
6. EMPOWERMENT

"It's that simple!"

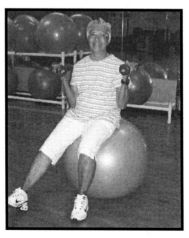

Maria, 82 years young, is an awesome athlete who is balanced.

Nora is trapped. Two hundred pounds overweight, she is a member of a popular diet program, one of many she has attempted to follow. Furthermore, she suffers from food allergies that appear as hives and come and go as unexpected as their cause. Every diet makes Nora feel less in control and more trapped. Most diet foods either fail to satisfy her or set off her allergy symptoms. With all of the weight she has to lose, she is starting to wonder if it's worth the effort. After all, the small changes she works hard for in five days can be totally wiped out with a day or two of a food binge. This is a pattern she has experienced her whole life. She once blamed it on school, and now she blames it on her demanding job. When she comes home from work, the last thing she wants to worry about is what to eat, how to prepare food, and what she can or can't have. She is convinced that those who are thin either live in a totally deprived state, or they are blessed with fast metabolisms that burn all the food they eat.

Natalie is free. She lives the six-step process. When I started working with Natalie, I think she was expecting a long list of what not to eat as well as a list of "Myrna" foods that enable me to stay lean and athletic. At less than five feet, Natalie's frame had difficultly carrying the extra 70 pounds she had put on. After 20 years of trying every diet program, shots, and medically supervised starvation programs, she had decided that being thin was just not her body type, because her body always went back to its old overweight self. At age 45, she had decided to accept herself and realize this was the body she was going to have, and that being fat was what her body wanted. She was further convinced that the only weight-loss programs that worked were the ones that had the good and bad list of foods, with a program that kept you accountable. Her past experiences had convinced her that she couldn't trust herself. Therefore, she was sure, that because the six-step program didn't focus on weight loss, it would not help her lose weight. Natalie wanted to be healthy more than she cared about being thin. She also wanted more energy. Like many, she was tired of being tired. That was six years ago. Her weight of 105 pounds is perfect for her frame. She has never felt as if she was on a diet. In fact, she claims she eats double the amounts of foods she use to eat when she was overweight.

What Makes Nora Different?

What is different about Nora, who struggles with an extra two hundred pounds, and Natalie, who enjoys her perfect body weight? The answer is: *the mind working <u>with</u> the body.* The key to success is to balance the body so you can affect the thought process, which is the root of the problem. Otherwise you have a brain-versus-body battle. You get there by educating yourself on how to do this rewire job through the six steps.

You won't find a diet plan in this book. Diet plans work only temporarily, if they work at all. No single food is ruled out. After all, no single food is the answer for total health, nor is it the reason for why you are overweight.

Nora believes (as you may) that it is about the external influences, the perfect diet program, the perfect body weight. What she (and maybe you) fail to see, is that living a healthy lifestyle is a part of your life, not a diet or special formula. It is about what is happening deep within your thoughts. It is about the mind and how to recondition that mind so that you will want to follow through on healthy behavior that will reinforce positive beliefs about you and the world around you. It is hard to recondition your mind if your body isn't on board. The six-step process worked for Natalie because it reconditioned her thoughts through a process that balanced her body.

Natalie's six steps are different now than when she first started. The point being that the foods that make up your six steps today, may be very different than the foods you grow to love. The six-step process will evolve as you do. As you become balanced and your body is able to regulate itself the internal battle disappears and you will be empowered to make healthier food choices.

The six steps remain the same now as they will fifty years from now.

There is no quick fix, and there is no magic formula. It is not about eating certain foods or not eating other foods. No, it is much simpler than that. It is about you and understanding how to unlock the process inside of you.

The six-step process will evolve with you, conditioning you each day for what you can handle for that day. Although the six steps remain the same, no one's six steps are identical, and none of us is a carbon copy of another.

"Let's get started so you can get started!"

THREE

FIRST STEP, WATER

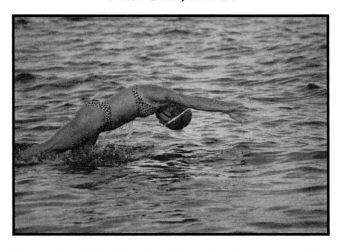

Myrna dives into a beach swim workout

Only Water Hydrates

When people think of hydration, most of the time they just think about quenching their thirst. Thirst is just a symptom that is warning us of a serious condition. Simply stated, hydration is a condition you choose to be in. It is black and white. You are either hydrated or dehydrated. The only thing that is grey is that you may think you are hydrated when you are actually chronically dehydrated. This may not seem like a big deal until I explain how damaging dehydration is to every cell in your body. Once again, this is a condition you choose, every day, by the food and liquid choices you make, not realizing the imbalances you create.

Water Doesn't Create Balance…Water *is* Balance

Any food or liquid we ingest creates and requires some type of action from the body, or in some cases reaction. Depending on the food and your current state, you could be better or worse for it. What happens with food or other liquids is that the body has a full-time job of trying to figure out how to break it down, use it, or store the unused portion. Once you eat or drink something, it becomes a balancing act. Let's take for example, sugar-loaded liquids such as lemonade, fruit punch or sweet tea. The body's reaction to these types of liquids is much different than plain water. High sugar liquids cause an excessive surge of the hormone, *insulin* to balance the imbalance you created from the excess sugar, which, in turn, causes you to feel tired and actually crave more sugar, which then causes weight gain. This is just one example of how water that has sugar added to it can affect hormonal balance, causing a domino effect of more imbalances, like obesity and fatigue. It isn't just limited to hormones. It affects bones, skin, major organs, and just about every cell in our body. They can all be affected by poor liquid choices.

Every time you put food or liquid in your body, you may be stepping onto a roller coaster of ups and downs. Your reaction to these substances can determine your state of mind, energy level, and overall health.

Water is Neutral

Everything we put into our body demands some type of chemical action, except pure water. Water is the only element that we put in our bodies that is neutral. There is no balancing act with water. Water by its very nature is balanced, which makes it very soothing for the body, which means it isn't an energy drain.

Water is the super daddy of balance, for the simple fact it doesn't create an imbalance. The problem is a lot of people add ingredients to their super daddy thinking it is better to have a sugar daddy, only to find out their sugar daddy creates all sorts of imbalances causing an unstable lifestyle. This isn't about some guy your daughter is dating, this is you...on liquid!

Water has less obvious benefits such as:

→ Plumps the cells which make you look younger.
→ Cleans the body of toxic waste.
→ Creates an environment for muscle movement.
→ Regulates the bowels.
→ Allows you to think clearly.
→ Increases metabolic function.

Proper hydration is not just about quenching your thirst. It is a condition you choose that allows for an optimum state of good health. If you drink only when you are thirsty, you already suffer from dehydration.

Research shows that as little as a 2 percent drop in body water weight can cause memory loss and difficulty in focusing on daily tasks. It can also trigger fatigue and muscle soreness. Those who suffer from back and joint pain have had relief from increasing water consumption. Even mild dehydration has shown to cause a sluggish metabolism. It is obvious that without water we cease to survive. It is the precursor for every bodily function.

Consumption of liquids other than water can actually cause dehydration. This happens with caffeinated beverages such as colas, teas, and energy drinks, as well as alcoholic beverages. You have to watch out for these sugar daddys! They will trick you into believing you are hydrated, as well as giving you a false sense of balance, robbing you of good health.

Liquids Other Than Water Can Cause Imbalance and Dehydration

The problem is that dehydration can occur without any indication. You may experience symptoms of dehydration and not even realize it is related to a lack of water. Since you may not be thirsty, you might not associate your headaches, constipation, muscle pain, skin irritations, foggy thoughts, and fatigue to a lack of water, especially if you are drinking liquids other than water that cause hormone surges, nervousness, or dehydration. So in your mind, you are sure you are hydrated because of that 32 ounce cola you consume every morning on your way to work, when actually the caffeine and the added mineral phosphorus are causing a dehydrated condition and calcium depletion. You end up asking yourself why your brain feels as if it is in a fog and your muscles lack motivation. Perhaps the two-hour buzz from the caffeine is worth spending the rest of the day cloaked in fatigue.

Soft Drinks Do More Than Dehydrate; They Cause Bone Loss

Considering that colas and diet colas are the preferred choice of beverage among youth and dieters, the imbalance that occurs from soft drinks that contain the mineral phosphorus needs mentioning. Phosphorus, a naturally occurring mineral that is found in colas, soft drinks and naturally occurs in most animal proteins, such as meat and cheese, causes calcium depletion. Here is how it works. The body maintains a perfect ratio of calcium to phosphorus in our blood, and when we disrupt this balance the body pulls calcium from the bones to maintain the ratio in the blood.

In other words, we cause a mild continual flow of calcium to seep from our bones into our blood to correct the imbalance we created when we consumed high concentrations of phosphorous.

Research shows that just one cola can have a negative effect, and when combined with caffeine, the effect is increased. We never feel these imbalances as they happen. Usually, the only indication of osteoporosis, (bone loss) is the unattractive slump you see in many middle age women, which is usually a precursor of the aches, pains and fractures that they may suffer years later.

Certain Diet Conditions Can Cause Imbalance and Dehydration

When you choose carbohydrate restriction, you are choosing a dehydrated condition. This is how many weight-loss programs can promise a 15-25 pound loss in 30 days. It would be virtually impossible to lose 20 pounds of body fat in 30 days, but totally possible to drop 25-30 pounds of water. Unfortunately, you may not feel thirsty as your cells shrivel up, and your muscles lack the hydration to adequately perform. Sometimes you may not associate your fatigue or afternoon headaches to the fact that you live a dehydrated lifestyle. Weight management through water loss is just a tricky form of dehydration, and can be very dangerous over a prolonged period of time.

If you exist on a low-carbohydrate diet, as soon as you eat one to two servings of carbohydrates, your body begins to hydrate. This hydration can cause one to two pounds of weight gain almost immediately, leading to the myth that carbohydrates make you fat!

Not so. Eliminating carbohydrates from your diet causes your body to go into a dehydrated state. Carbohydrates keep the hydration in your body, it is what helps make the water stay with you. Just drinking water alone may not be enough to hydrate a person who restricts carbohydrates, it is as if the water goes right through them instead of sticking with them.

Dangerously restricting carbohydrates causes fluid imbalances that cause water loss within the muscles, which limits muscle movement. Muscles need water to move

People who are usually mislead into believing carbohydrate restriction is the solution to weight loss fall into this trap. Low-carbohydrate lifestyle leads to a low activity because of the negative effect it has on muscles.

The Water-Muscle Formula:

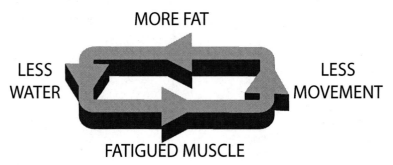

MORE FAT

LESS
WATER

LESS
MOVEMENT

FATIGUED MUSCLE

If muscles are not well hydrated or fueled properly they are unable to move. In fact, poorly hydrated muscles make joints and muscles feel achy, which makes it tough to move around, and as you can guess, the less mobile the more fat.

Carbohydrates provide the needed fuel and water for muscles. That is why they are called: carbo-HYDRATES. (carbo- means fuel, and hydrate means water). High protein, carbohydrate restrictive diets cause a domino effect of ill health such as bone loss, joint and muscle pain, and lack of desire to be active. This will be explained in more detail in the protein step.

How Much Water Do You Need?

The average person requires 64 ounces or 8, 8 ounce glasses per day of liquid. One could also calculate this requirement based on half of his/her body weight in ounces. That can seem an insurmountable challenge especially if you are struggling with obesity. It would be almost impossible to try and meet the quota of 12-15 glasses of water for someone carrying 70-100 pounds of excess weight. Pure water is what is recommended to keep balance. Most people drink half their consumption of liquid from tea, cola's and coffee and even then fall short of meeting their hydration requirement. Research supports dehydration is a common condition among obese individuals. Just increasing to eight glasses a day can be a great challenge and is a major hurdle. Sometimes it can take a while before your body accepts it as part of your lifestyle. Once you get into the habit of drinking water, it gets easier. Perhaps because it makes you feel better, and your body begins to crave it.

STEP ONE – WATER

1. Drink 64 ounces or 8, 8 ounce glasses of water daily.

2. Avoid sugary drinks.

3. Avoid sodas.

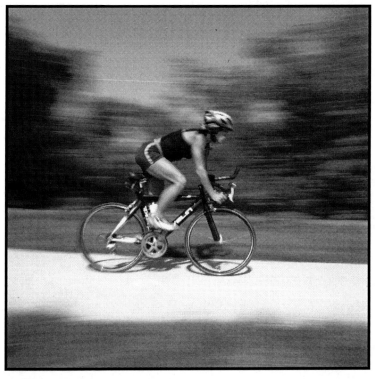

Myrna zips along

FOUR

PROTEIN-FIBER COMBINATIONS

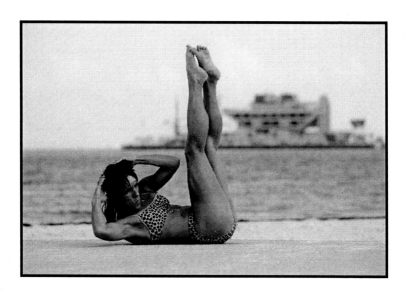

Just Two Meals Away From Making a Difference

You will find all six steps are important in bringing you into balance, but the step that has the most impact to immediately change your body chemistry is protein and fiber foods eaten in the **right amounts**, at the **right time**. In fact, when protein and fiber are properly combined, you are only two meals away from total balance or total imbalance. Just two meals away from being in an addiction or totally free from food's hold over you. In other words, if you can educate yourself and become pretty good at knowing how to work this magic combination, the internal battle is gone!

When You Remove the Internal Turmoil, You Remove the Addiction

Now, let's imagine you with no food addiction. What if you could pass by your favorite foods and not have them call your name. In fact, what if your entire pantry was full of food that normally would cause such an internal unrest that you wouldn't dare tempt yourself? What if you could be two meals away from this being you? What would you be like if food didn't matter? What if you never got hungry, and eating broccoli provided as much comfort and joy as German chocolate cake or warm-soft buttered bread? If this were you over time, any excess weight would melt away, and the best part is you wouldn't have to stay on a diet because it wasn't a diet that got you there. Then you would be one of those naturally thin people who get to eat anything and as much as you desire, because when you change your chemistry, you change your desire. It is that simple and all of the tools you need to make it easy are right here.

When people fall off the wagon from days or weeks of food binging, a feeling of doom and gloom hangs over them. To get back on track can mean weeks, maybe months, of dieting, which usually means food deprivation and excessive exercise. What if all that could go away? What if you knew you were only two meals, not two months, from being back to the place you need to be? This is not about a <u>diet</u>. It is about a <u>life</u> you choose, a state of <u>being</u> you choose to be in.

Knowing how to combine protein and fiber in the right amounts at the right times has the most immediate impact of putting you in that place. All that is required are two meals of the right combinations, and your body chemistry will snap into place. Just like that. Conversely, you are also that close to creating an imbalance and once again being a victim of food.

Even if you choose foods that may not have the highest quality, you will still be free of food addiction and have an increase in energy. Although eventually everyone who follows the six steps evolves to higher quality foods, at first they stick with foods they like and are familiar with. This is wonderful because the six steps will meet you wherever you are in your journey, and will make a huge impact in your life.

Once the protein-fiber combinations are working for you, it becomes a whole lot easier to exercise, because you will have a lot more energy. Once you have more energy, you will feel like moving around, which results in a leaner, healthier you. The six steps become a domino effect, and the more you define them, the stronger and more defined you become.

The six steps are not about being perfect; they're about being you. In order for them to work for you, an education and some basic tools are required. Don't worry; I am not going to ask you to focus on any particular food lists of what you can and can't have, because it isn't about the foods. It is all about you around food, which makes this the last book you'll ever buy on dieting, and one of many books on health.

"*Are you ready to discover how protein and fiber can rock your world?*"

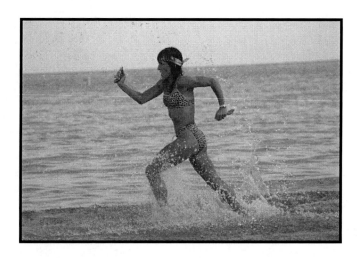

Myrna water running in St. Petersburg, Florida

FIVE

WHAT YOU NEED TO KNOW ABOUT PROTEIN

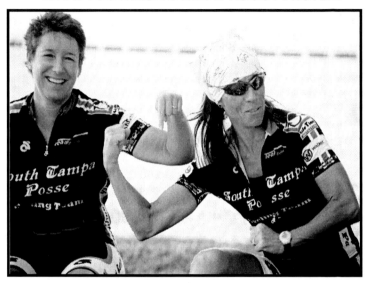

Lynnie trying not to laugh too loud over Myrna's massive muscles.

Why Should I Care About Protein?

Regardless if you're in it for your health, or just looking to drop a few extra pounds, protein foods can be the golden gate to health or the door to the abyss. Protein used wisely can deliver one heck of a body, but irresponsible consumption can put you at risk for certain cancers, heart disease, overall fatigue, and really rotten health.

Your body uses protein every minute of the day. Everything your body does to keep you alive requires protein. That includes all your cells, vital organs, and hormones. Even your brain is made from protein. Proteins are the body's building materials responsible for repairing and building that fleshy cage you live in.

The only access we have to certain vital proteins is through our diet, and if you don't eat the right combinations in the right amounts at the best time, you are in big trouble! You won't drop dead immediately, but you'll have a miserable lingering existence.

It helps to know what foods have protein in them, but it doesn't stop there. You still need to know how to optimally balance these vital nutrients. Protein is what most diets use to accelerate weight loss, but at the cost of creating a protein imbalance that leaves you in a bigger mess than before the diet. You are temporarily thinner but with a whole new set of problems of which you are unaware.

Animal foods and animal food by-products have the highest concentration of protein. These include meats like chicken, turkey, fish, hamburger, steak, and by-products such as, eggs, milk, and cheese. Plant foods also have protein such as: soy, beans, nuts, seed and grains, and to a lesser extent, some fruits and vegetables.

How to Balance Protein.

Many times you don't associate ill health or weight gain with a protein imbalance, especially if you think you are eating healthy foods. Most people unintentionally have a protein imbalance and are unaware that this could be the cause of excess weight, food addictions, overall fatigue and poor health. The American belief is that protein is healthy, and an excess is even better. This is not correct.

The truth is: protein is healthy, but only when properly balanced. The fear of weight gain and carbohydrate consumption has many of us confused as to what is this proper balance.

THE FOUR FACTORS FOR PROTEIN BALANCE

1. The Right <u>Amount</u> of Protein
2. The Right <u>Combinations</u> of Proteins
3. The Right <u>Timing</u> of Protein
4. Using Proteins for their <u>Designated Purpose</u>

1. The Right Amount of Protein

Approximately every nine months, most cells in the body die off and are remade, (except bone, which takes longer). What this means is that, in one year's time, you have the opportunity to create an awesome body or really mess it up.

Deprive your body of protein, and it improvises by eating away healthy muscle tissue or vital organs.

Since the body absolutely needs protein to survive, it doesn't wait for you to feed it the right amount at the right time. There is a rich source of protein in muscle tissue that your body will resort to using when the diet is lacking. You are not aware as your body is eating away healthy muscle tissue for the needed protein nutrients. You won't feel it, because there is no pain or indication that this is happening. Feeding on your own muscle tissue and possibly vital organs for nutrients is not a good thing! If you do not properly balance protein, this is exactly what happens.

Lose Weight, But Don't Lose Muscle

Let's suppose you are trying to lose weight, and you decide to speed up the weight-loss process by eating mostly fruits and vegetables and not eating enough protein to support your body weight. What if some advertisement has convinced you to do a three-day fast of special weight-loss juices? Most likely you will lose weight, but part of the weight loss will be lean healthy muscle tissue. Why? Because your body was forced to eat your muscles for the needed nutrients. This makes it the dumbest weight loss program ever—eating away the only thing that will keep you lean—muscle tissue!

Don't Eat Muscle

Muscle tissue is something you work hard for. It only happens through movement. And the less you move, the less you have. If you chose to eat away muscle, the only way to get it back is through movement. You do not eat your way into a muscular body. Any muscle tissue your body was forced to eat for nutrients is lost forever, and any excess weight you gain after your diet will come back as fat, not muscle.

So fasting or not eating enough protein makes you fatter. You may lose weight initially, but the real question is: are you losing fat or muscle? If you eat away muscle tissue, in the long run, you set yourself up to be overweight. The more overweight you are, the slower your metabolism, which makes it much harder every diet cycle. The last thing you want to do is eat away muscle tissue or compromise vital organs, so it is important to know exactly how much protein you need to maintain what you already have. How much protein you need is determined by how much you weigh. It doesn't matter if it is fat or muscle, the body needs a certain amount of protein to maintain the weight you carry around. Remember protein's role is to maintain and repair all of the cells in your body and build new ones. If you lose weight, then there is less of you to maintain, and the protein requirement will be less.

A quick and easy way to calculate your daily protein requirement is to divide your current weight in half, this number will be the amount of protein grams you need daily. This is only slightly higher than the exact calculation of multiplying your current body weight by 0.4.

Know Your Protein Requirement

Body weight x 0.4 = __   minimum daily protein grams required

Example:

200 pounds x 0.4 =   <u>80</u>   minimum daily protein grams required

---

Based on this formula a 200 pound person needs 80 grams of protein per day to maintain their protein balance. Consuming less than 80 grams per day would not be adequate to maintain a 200 pound person; therefore the body would resort to cannibalism.

Physical Activity Requires More Protein

Physical activity breaks down muscle tissue more than being sedentary, which means your protein requirements increase with exercise. The last thing you want to do is spend one-to-two hours in a gym and then have your body eat away muscle tissue you've worked so hard to gain.

The more time spent in exercise and level of intensity, the greater the need for more protein. Just one-to-two hours per day of physical activity can result in a 15-20 percent increase in protein. This seems like a lot, but actually it works out to be only 20-30 grams more for the whole day. That's less than 3 ounces of chicken or one cup of cottage cheese.

No exercise
Current weight _____ x .4 _____ protein grams

Exercising 0-1 hours per day:
Current weight _____ x .5-.6 = _____ protein grams

Exercising 1-3 hours per day
Current weight _____ x .6-.8 = _____ protein grams

Exercising > 3 hours per day
Current weight _____ x .8-1.5 = _____ protein grams

If you exercise anywhere from one-to-two hours per day, then multiply your body weight by 0.5 - 0.6, which is still pretty close to the rough estimation of half your body weight.

Minimum
200 pounds x 0.6 = _120_ daily protein grams required

Let's assume this 200-pound person engages in a two-hour exercise program. This increases the protein requirement by an additional 40 grams per day. Which is like adding two glasses of milk and 4 ounces chicken for the entire day.

Professional Athletes Require More Protein

There are some people who really hit it hard for four-to-six hours per day, increasing their protein requirement to as much as 0.8 – 1.0 their body weight.

200 pounds x 0.8 = <u>160</u> minimum daily protein grams required

What is a Protein Gram?

Grams are just a measurement that tells us how much of something is in a certain weight. In this case, we use grams to tell us how much fiber, protein carbohydrates and fat are in food. A food label is required to list how many grams of each are in one serving.

All packaged foods sitting on your grocery stores shelves are required by law to have a label on them that tells you the amount of protein it has in one serving. Processed packaged food can be a real bag of surprises, which is why the government requires a label in the first place. That means you need to understand how to read it.

Nutrition Facts

Serving Size 1/2 cup (about 82g)
Servings Per Container 8

Amount Per Serving

Calories 200   Calories from Fat 130

% Daily Value*

Total Fat 14g	**22%**
Saturated Fat 9g	**45%**
Trans Fat 0g	
Cholesterol 55mg	**18%**
Sodium 40mg	**2%**
Total Carbohydrate 17g	**6%**
Dietary Fiber 1g	**4%**
Sugars 14g	
Protein 3g	

Vitamin A 10%	•	Vitamin C 0%
Calcium 10%	•	Iron 6%

*Percent Daily Values are based on a 2,000 calorie diet. Your daily values may be higher or lower depending on your calorie needs:

		Calories:	2,000	2,500
Total Fat	Less than		65g	80g
Saturated Fat	Less than		20g	25g
Cholesterol	Less than		300mg	300 mg
Sodium	Less than		2,400mg	2,400mg
Total Carbohydrate			300g	375g
Dietary Fiber			25g	30g

Calories per gram:
        Fat 9 • Carbohydrate 4 • Protein 4

It is worth it for you to find out how many grams of protein are in your favorite foods. I have listed a few protein foods that don't have labels.

Food	Protein
1 cup beans	15 grams
3 oz. meat, chicken, fish	22 grams
1 egg	7 grams
1 oz. cheese	7 grams
½ cup soy-nuts	10 grams
½ cup peanuts	6 grams

How Do Protein Grams Measure Up With Calories?

On average, approximately 12 to 20 percent of your total daily calories should come from protein. In calorie language, this means if you consume 2,000 calories per day, only about 300-400 calories will come from protein.

In food language, this works out to be 80-100 grams of protein, which translates to 6 ounces of chicken, 1 cup of beans and rice, and one serving yogurt, for the entire day! If you have calculated the amount of protein needed for your body weight, you will find that it is a relatively small percentage based on the total number of calories you consume.

Too Much Protein Can Make You Fat and Unhealthy.

What should seem very obvious to you is that we need a lot less protein than what is currently being advocated by most diets, eating establishments, and the food industry. Americans eat two to three times their daily requirement of protein because they don't know how to properly balance protein and are unaware this can cause obesity and poor health.

What can be confusing for a lot of people is that although protein is healthy and does a lot of great good for the body, an excess of protein can cause havoc.

What Happens With Excess Protein?

Once the body uses the amount of protein that is needed to build and repair, any excess protein is stored as body fat. I'm sure you've had diet books sell you on the idea that consuming excess protein is ideal, because the body uses protein for fuel instead of nasty carbohydrates that are usually to blame for obesity. Yes, the body is able to use protein for fuel, but only if there are no other foods available, as in the case when carbohydrates are restricted or eliminated.

Converting protein into fuel is a laborious task that strains the liver, kidneys, and causes muscle fatigue. The only nasty thing here is how you will feel. Any excess protein you consume over your daily requirement will turn to fat, unless you force your body to use it as fuel, in which case will cause another protein imbalance where protein is not used for its designated purpose, which we will discuss in more detail later.

2. The Right combinations of Protein

Having the right amount of protein is important, but making sure you have the right combinations of proteins is equally as important. In fact, not having the right combinations of protein has the same effect as not getting enough.

How it Works

Since the body needs protein for every second we are alive, nature provided a **protein reserve,** a special pool of proteins that the body can access at any time. Otherwise, we would have to eat protein every minute of the day! This protein reserve is where the body stores the protein units called amino acids. There are 22 amino acid units in all, and they must all be readily available in your reserve to work properly. Just one missing amino acid can throw the entire reserve out of balance, and the body will be forced to go to muscle tissue and vital organs for the essential amino acids. The body treats poor-quality protein in the same way that it treats a lack of protein.

Bottom line:
It is important to make sure you get the right amount of protein as well as the right quality of proteins. Otherwise, you risk having a protein deficiency.
Protein cannot do its job unless all amino acids are available in the right amount.

Know Which Foods Have All The Amino Acids.

Although all protein foods have a certain number of amino acids, not all of them have <u>all</u> the 22 amino acids you need to keep your reserve healthy. This means you have to be smart how to combine or include certain proteins.

Protein foods that have all the amino acids in them are called **complete proteins**. These proteins are the complete package. Include these in your diet, and your reserve will be balanced providing all the amino acids the body needs to keep you operating optimally.

<u>**Complete proteins**</u> come from animal foods and animal by-products, such as milk, cheese, eggs, chicken, fish, and meat. One of the few plant foods that are complete is Soy which includes soy products, such as soybeans, tofu, and soy milk.

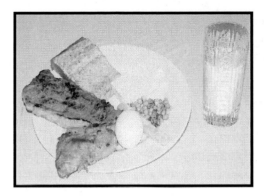

This picture is an example of complete proteins: Soynuts, Chicken, Egg, Steak, Fish, Tofu, and Milk

Protein foods that are missing one or two amino acids are called incomplete proteins. **<u>Incomplete proteins</u>** come from plant foods, such as beans, nuts, seeds, grains, and vegetables. These foods need to be combined with each other or complete proteins in order to provide all the right amino acids.

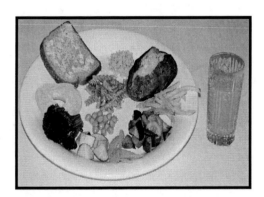

This picture is an example of incomplete proteins: Potato, French Fries, Vegetables, Fruit, Beans, Bagel, Bread, and Orange Juice

Incomplete plant proteins need to be combined with each other, or a complete protein food included in the mix, to have all of the essential amino acids that are needed for the body to build and repair itself. Otherwise, incomplete proteins are ineffective protein sources, because the body won't have all 22 amino acids available. If the body goes to the protein reserve and finds only 20 or 21 amino acids, and just one essential amino acid is missing, then you have created an imbalance, and the body will search for the missing amino acid in your own healthy tissue

The Total Protein Package

If you choose not to eat any animal proteins, and you are unable to eat soy proteins, you will need to know how to combine incomplete plant protein foods with other incomplete plant protein foods that happen to have the missing amino acids. As in the case with beans and rice or peanut butter and bread, all of these foods are incomplete proteins by themselves, but when combined together, they create the total protein package.

Beans have all but two amino acids, and rice has the two amino acids that beans are missing. This happens with most plant foods except soy. Soy is one of the few plant proteins that is complete.

Another way to keep the protein reserve balanced is to include a complete protein in the entire meal mix.

A daily diet that includes some type of animal proteins or soy protein stops you from going crazy trying to figure out how to combine incomplete proteins. Current studies support that as long as you consume a complete protein or maintain proper combining of incomplete proteins with in a 12- to 24-hour period, the amino acid reserve should have an adequate balance of all 22 amino acids. Even a small number of complete proteins in the whole diet mix make the protein reserve balanced. That explains why underdeveloped countries with a scarce supply of animal foods include soybeans in a vegetarian mix, so that entire meal becomes complete with all the essential amino acids available to maintain a healthy body.

Balanced Reserve Saves Muscle

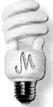 A balanced protein reserve means you will have a leaner body, because you are healthier and your body isn't eating away muscle tissue.

Let's suppose you have cereal with milk for breakfast, and a large bowl of vegetables and rice for lunch. The complete protein from the milk at breakfast should keep your amino acid reserve balanced for most of the day. (Just keep in mind you still have to maintain an adequate amount of protein for your weight.) If you go more than a day of eating incomplete proteins, then you have a big problem. This can happen when people believe crazy diets of single foods will make them healthier or thinner.

Regardless of all the health benefits you get from eating plant foods, if you don't understand how to keep your amino acid reserve adequately supplied, you are not healthy. It doesn't matter how many vitamins, minerals and enzymes you consume with healthy vegetables and fruits; you can still have a sub-optimal protein balance. It is the same as trying to build a house with all the needed materials except the nails. Even if you have the lumber and the kitchen sink, not much is happening without the nails. Protein works the same way. You can have plenty of it, but if you don't have the *right combinations*, not much will happen.

Incomplete plant proteins when combined together make complete protein

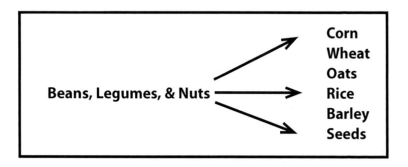

**Note for vegetarians.
If you are interested in living a strict vegetarian lifestyle with select proteins, please make an appointment with a registered dietician who can advise you on menu details.

Don't be Fooled by Food Labels!

As you read the label of a can of beans, it looks pretty good, doesn't it? You believe it has 8 grams of protein per serving as the label claims, but in reality it is 8 grams of protein *when combined with rice*. Food labels can be misleading because they do not tell us if the protein is incomplete or complete.

Peanut butter on a celery stick, or by the spoonful, is an incomplete protein. The missing amino acids that would allow peanut butter to be complete are found in the wheat grain in bread, which makes a peanut butter sandwich a complete protein food.

Oat cereal is missing a few amino acids, but combining it with milk, which has all the amino acids, makes the cereal a complete protein meal. Once again, it is not a problem if you eat smart and know how to properly combine incomplete proteins or include complete proteins in your foods at some time within the day. Each meal is not as significant as your total daily diet when it comes to protein combinations.

Combine the Right Proteins

Animal Food   **+**   **Any Food**
(Complete Protein)

OR

Plant Food   **+**   **Plant Food**
(Beans, Legumes, Nuts)   (Corn, wheat, oats, rice, etc.)
                             or Animal Food

=

Complete Protein (all 22 amino acids)

Emily wants to be thin at any cost

Emily was so fearful of getting fat that food became the enemy. Her eating and exercise rituals included low-calorie vegetables and long exercise sessions. What Emily didn't realize is that thin and lean are not the same. And by not allowing her body the essential amino acids, she was compromising valuable muscle tissue as well as her health. Emily did not understand the importance of keeping her proteins balanced. She was focused only on being thin, which meant a smaller size even if it meant losing muscle.

Perfect bodies are in reach for all of us, but you cannot have a prefect body that is depleted in nutrients, and you cannot have a perfect body if you have imbalances. Perfect bodies are strong, lean healthy machines that look and feel awesome and come in many different sizes and shapes! Protein plays a significant role in allowing our bodies to keep the muscle, and not knowing how to balance proteins compromises your body's muscle-to-fat ratio.

In other words, when you compromise your body's ability to repair muscle, it is the same as asking the body to eat away at the only hope you have of being lean. Because muscles that aren't fed properly can't be used adequately, this leads to atrophied muscle marbled with fat. Being lean is all about having muscles that are fed properly. For Emily to be lean, she'd have to eat a lot more food, ensuring that her muscles had the right fuel for exercise, and also the proper balance of proteins. She could then have a fit body that weighed more, but was leaner.

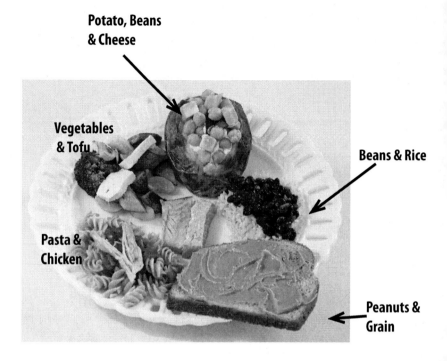

Potato, Beans & Cheese

Vegetables & Tofu

Beans & Rice

Pasta & Chicken

Peanuts & Grain

Combining Incomplete Protein to make a Complete Protein

3. The Right Timing of Protein

The Body Only Absorbs Small Amounts of Protein at One Time.

Just because you've eaten your daily requirement of protein as well as included complete proteins in your diet doesn't mean you have protein balance. The third major factor in balancing protein is *proper timing.*

Every minute of the day the human body is constantly creating new cells to replace old ones. As mentioned previously, amino acids are the building materials that the cells use to make the repairs. How healthy or how strong you are depends on how well the body repairs itself, which is why the amino acid reserve is so critical.

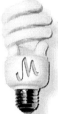

Protein Absorbtion
Your body cannot absorb large quantities of protein at one time, so you can't eat all your daily protein requirements at one meal.

For most people, the body can only absorb 20-30 grams of protein during a single meal. If your daily requirement of protein is 60 grams for the entire day, (refer to the formula; body weight x .4), you would need 15-20 grams of protein for meals, and 6-8 grams of protein for snacks.

The most efficient way to replenish the amino acid reserve is to eat smaller portions of protein throughout the day

Let's suppose you eat a whole roasted chicken for dinner. Your body would still use only one chicken thigh (approx. 25 grams) to build and repair itself, then store the excess as body fat. You can force your body to use protein for fuel, lessening the chance it will be stored as fat, but this is not utilizing protein for its designated purpose, and it creates further imbalances, which we will discuss in more detail later.

4. Using Proteins for Their Designated Purpose

Utilizing proteins for purposes other than what they are designated, causes a protein imbalance. Protein imbalances make you fatter by slowing down your metabolism.

The last significant factor in balancing protein is to use it for the role for which it was intended. Amino acids have a designated purpose, to build and repair the body. The body is able to use protein for fuel. This is what the body does in cases of survival where protein is the only food source available. Otherwise humans may not have survived the last million years. Just because amino acids have the ability to multi-task doesn't make it optimal for your health. In fact, just the opposite is true. Asking amino acids to be used as fuel puts you at risk for poor health, weight gain, and debilitating fatigue.

Excess Protein is Bad

When the body uses excess protein as fuel, it expels uric acid in your urine, sweat, and even your lungs. This explains the bad breath for people on high protein diets. Secreting high amounts of acidic waste is a trigger for other health problems, such as gout, osteoporosis, chronic fatigue, impaired immune function, and kidney and liver stress. This type of high protein imbalance creates an acidic environment that results in dehydration, muscle fatigue, vulnerability to minor colds and infections, and, as research shows, a high correlation with certain cancers and heart disease.

Don't Use Protein for Fuel

Let's suppose you are on a diet of high protein and low carbohydrate foods. You are told this is the quickest method for weight loss, and those carbohydrates foods such as bread, beans, and potatoes make you fat. When carbohydrate foods are eliminated, the body's only options for fuel are protein and fat. Keep in mind that proteins were not designed to be used to fuel our muscles. This is a job best done by carbohydrates, although protein can be converted into glucose (sugar) for the muscles when there is no other option. If muscles don't have glucose, you literally become dead in your tracks! And, since the body can't wait for you to get smart, it does what it must to survive!

The process of using proteins for fuel can happen within a few days of consuming excessive amounts of protein and restricting carbohydrates. The body has to go through a chemical process to make these proteins available for fuel. As already mentioned, it isn't an easy task. It weakens the immune system and causes strain on major organs, resulting in excess amounts of uric waste in your urine, leaving your cells dehydrated and acidic.

Dehydration and acidity cause a domino effect for other major imbalances that can cause serious illness. It is very simple. Muscles need water, and when they are dehydrated, fatigue sets in, and your entire mineral balance is thrown off. Your cells shrivel up. They are thirsty. But you don't feel thirsty; you feel thin. That's right. You lose a lot of water weight, and you look 10-15 pounds thinner, and everyone tells you how fantastic you look. Forget the fact you're killing yourself, and you feel more rotten than the morning garbage. You are convinced this is the secret to thinness. Every diet program knows this chemical process will make you thinner by causing dehydration. This dehydrated condition gives the dieter a false sense of weight loss.

This is a trap! The truth is, you can never stay thin this way, because your body isn't balanced, and, believe me, it will swing you in the other direction. This is called yo-yo dieting. Being thin is not the answer. Being lean is. Lean happens when muscles lose fat. Thin happens when you drop weight.

Lean happens when muscles are toned and tight. This can't happen when muscles are dehydrated and unable to move. You can't get toned and tight muscles unless you move them, and you can't move them unless they are well fed and hydrated!

High Protein Diets Cause Weight Gain...Don't Fall for This Trap

If your body is dehydrated from a high protein diet, the first bite of a starch or sugar of any kind will re-hydrate your body, and you will gain one to two pounds in the process. Think of how depressing it would be if you gained two pounds from eating one slice of bread or enjoying a few bites of dessert. Calorically, this would be impossible and should never happen, but if you are dehydrated, this is your body's way of fixing an imbalanced protein dehydrated condition.

Water hydrates more effectively when carbohydrates are included. If you are on a carbohydrate restricted diet and eat carbs, your body will immediately hydrate. With one bread or cake binge, a person could gain five to eight pounds of water, feeling and looking bloated and fat. This is mostly water weight, but it causes other addictive triggers, creating hormonal imbalances that make you feel tired, promote fat storage, and increase your desire for more sugar.

When the first opportunity arises, the body will binge on sugar to balance out the depleted carbohydrate reserve. In other words, the body finds opportunities to binge. The internal battle that we spoke about earlier will keep playing in your brain, and your body will make you want foods that you are trying to stay away from. When protein and carbohydrates are not properly balanced, food addiction is inevitable, and you won't be able to stay away from the foods that cause the problem. Learn how to balance your body, and you will no longer be the victim of the diet trap. Proper protein balance is the first step to total balance.

Excess Amounts of Protein Can Actually Inhibit the Ability to Build More Muscle and Lose Excess Fat!

A big myth is that protein foods build muscle. This is an exaggerated truth. The only way to build muscle is to move it! It is the result of physical activity that causes muscle strength and size. Protein foods repair the muscles that have been worked, but first you have to work. The result of hard work is what makes muscles leaner, stronger, and healthier.

Wrong protein combinations and timing sabotage Don's efforts

Donald has always struggled with his weight. He was obese as a child, and swore he would never relive those days. Still, he fights a 10- to 12-pound weight fluctuation and claims he can gain 5-10 pounds in one weekend. This is hard to imagine, considering that he exercises approximately one to two hours every day. Don lacks the muscular physique that one would expect from a guy who is diligent about lifting weights three to four times a week, and runs a weekly average of 20 miles.

He came to me for advice as to how to achieve more definition in his muscles. After reviewing his program, I realized Don's problem wasn't his workouts, but his diet. Although he ate healthy food, he didn't eat the right combinations of protein at the right times, and he wasn't using protein for its designated purpose.

Don ate only fruit until noon, and the rest of the day he ate vegetables with rice, and drank a lot of diet sodas. He consumed most of his protein in the evenings. It was easier for him to cook a half a chicken at night than try and mess with it during the day. He was afraid to eat too much during the day, because it made him feel tired and bloated. He said that the weekends were his reward for staying on his diet and exercise program, but found he would eat more than he should Saturdays and Sundays, which resulted in a few extra pounds Monday morning. That gain, of course, perpetuated the same Monday-Friday diet cycle. Donald knew he could make improvements, but felt most of the time he ate healthy, low calorie meals, which is why he couldn't understand why he was struggling with excess weight gain.

Don was a slave to his Monday-through-Friday routine. This method of eating had kept his weight down for several years, but he had slowly gained weight, and couldn't lose 15 pounds, He thought maybe his age was a factor, and wondered if perhaps he should accept the added pounds.

I assured him it was less about his age, and more about his lifestyle. Don's body was eating away the muscle mass he was working so hard to build during the day, because he wasn't supplying adequate protein to build and repair his muscle tissue after a hard day at the gym. When he finally did eat most of his protein, his body needed only a small amount, approximately a quarter of what he was eating. Don was eating half a roasted chicken thinking he was supplying his body with all the needed protein for the day, when his body only needed a drumstick.

Once Don understood that the body only absorbs and utilizes small protein portions at one time, he began to spread his protein quantities throughout the day. This improved his protein balance and helped control his blood sugar, which stopped the tired feeling after lunch. Don also learned that carbohydrates have their own balancing act, and once he practiced proper food balance, there was less urge to binge on the weekends because he felt more satisfied. Most important, his body became leaner and more muscular. Don's food balance was reflected in the energy he had throughout the day, as well as his workouts, where he was able to push harder resulting in muscle gain.

Summary

The right <u>amount</u> of protein
Body weight = _____ grams of protein required daily

The right <u>combinations</u> of protein
Complete proteins vs. Incomplete proteins

The right <u>timing</u> of protein
The body absorbs small quantities, 15–35 grams per meal and 8–15 grams per snack.

The <u>proper use</u> of protein
Use proteins for their designated purpose.

SIX

FIBER-CARBOHYDRATE BALANCE

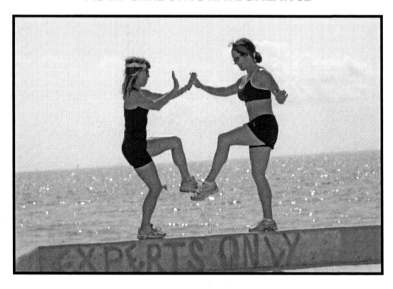

Whitney, (right), lost fat, gained muscle, proved balance is possible.

Carbohydrates Do Not Make You Fat

A common belief among many people is that carbohydrates make us fat, and eliminating or restricting them solves the problem. First of all, let's clear up some myths. Contrary to what you have heard, carbohydrates do not make you fat. Excess food of any kind makes you fat! Carbohydrates are energy foods that make you more active, and being more active results in a leaner body. The problem is that people do not know how to balance carbohydrates, which leads to food addictions, resulting in craving forbidden food that we know we shouldn't have but cannot resist.

The Forbidden Food

> *If you struggle with your weight, food addiction is the largest contributing factor as to why you can't seem to stay on a healthy diet and are unable to control yourself around food.*

Carbohydrates are frequently referred to as the forbidden foods – the ones that always seem to give us immediate, immense pleasure, only to make us feel worse afterwards. Maybe you have control over everything else in your life, and food is something you choose to ignore. After all, food is the center of entertainment, pleasure, and fulfillment. And don't we all deserve to enjoy life? The problem is not the food, but your feelings toward it. Carbohydrates do not just jump inside your body; you're the one who puts them there. You don't have to have a serious weight problem to be obsessed with food. You don't have to be overweight to have food make you crazy!

Food addiction doesn't discriminate. Hereditary tendencies, education level, and strong character play no part in who is affected. Food addiction can happen to anyone at any time. It is a result of the imbalances that we impose on ourselves from a lack of not knowing what it means to be balanced.

> *Food addiction is caused by carbohydrate and fiber imbalances that force the body to desire foods you don't want, but find irresistible.*

Some Food Manufacturers Aren't Helping

Food addiction sells products, which is a huge motivator for the food industry. It is hard to really know if the food industry purposely sells food-addictive products, but it is a fact that their wallets become fatter right along with our bodies. I think it is much easier for them to blame our lack of self control rather than their food.

How many times have you heard that being overweight means lack of self control, being irresponsible or lazy? If this were true, then why are registered dieticians, nurses, physicians, exercise trainers and highly educated successful people struggling with their weight? These professionals are highly motivated, responsible, and the very nature of their professions requires long, intense hours, showing no signs of laziness. What is really the underlining cause?

Even the most educated, self-motivated individuals have a hard time fighting food addiction. This is not about a lack of willpower. It is about the chemical state we put ourselves in unknowingly. Most people don't realize they have a food addiction. These are the same people who haven't really put the food puzzle together yet. They don't understand that packaged food is a commodity in the marketplace, just like oil, gold, and other products, and its sole purpose is to make money. It is a lot less expensive for food companies to feed addicts than people who eat healthy, balanced meals.

> *This book will show you how to unlock the rules of protein and fiber balance that will change your life.*

When Does the Addiction Stop?

When you are a victim of food addiction, you are unable to make good food choices, even if you want to. If food addiction was eliminated, imagine what a disaster it would be for the food industry. In America, we live in a hostile food environment where food is less about quality of life, and more about pleasure and addiction. This country has developed a multi-billion dollar industry that makes money from your addiction, then creates a temporary diet solution that generates billions of dollars, and by its very design, cycles you back into the addiction. Seldom are we controlled by celery, carrots, or a huge uncontrollable urge for a big bowl of broccoli.

Food addiction stops when you can live life in the six steps outlined in this book. Part of the six-step process is knowing how protein and fiber, in the **right amounts**, at the **right time** with the **right combinations,** can chemically change your body, which ultimately affects your thoughts**.**

What is Fiber?

Think of fiber as nature's packaging. It is what holds the carbohydrate material inside the plant. An example of nature's packaging would be the skin on the apple, or the outside barrier of a grain, which is called bran.

What is a Carbohydrate?

Carbohydrates are the starchy matter that is webbed inside all plants. Some plants, such as beans and grains, have more starchy matter than others, and plants, like spinach and broccoli, have less. The starchy filling in most plant foods is usually sweeter than the fiber, which is why food manufacturers remove and discard the fiber from most plant foods and sell it separately. When carbohydrates are eaten by themselves, you are on a slippery slope of food addiction, and you will consume double the calories than if the fiber had remained.

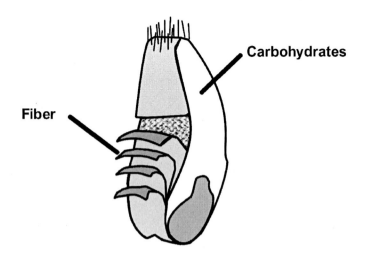

Where do Fiber and Carbohydrates Come From?

Fiber and carbohydrates are both found naturally in plants. Foods that come from plants are vegetables, fruits, seeds, nuts, beans, and grains. It is hard to tell if you are eating a plant when the food industry has replaced nature's packaging with their own. It's hard to think of a cookie as once being from a plant. The fact is that most foods on your grocery store shelf may have come from a plant at one time, but processing removed the fiber, which is the first assault in creating a chemical imbalance that causes the domino effect I mentioned before, and will explain later in more detail. A good rule of thumb is: If you can't eat the package, you shouldn't eat the food.

Fiber is found only in plants. Animal foods, such as meat, chicken, cheese, milk, and eggs, do not have fiber. Some animal foods, such as milk and yogurt, have a small number of carbohydrates, but you won't find fiber in these foods, unless man has artificially added it. This doesn't mean you shouldn't eat it. It may actually be a better choice to choose the artificially added fiber than not. Keep in mind that the fibers found in nature are always the best.

How do Fiber and Carbohydrates Work Together?

Unless man has removed the fiber, plant foods in their natural form, such as bananas, apples, beans, and oats, start out with fiber and carbohydrates combined. Once we eat these foods, our body breaks them down, and they go their separate ways. Fiber is the part of the plant wall that gets left behind in the intestinal tract, creating intestinal balance and cleans the body of toxic waste. Carbohydrates are absorbed into the blood, providing energy for the muscles. Although they both are responsible for two very different but important jobs, when eaten together they create balance.

In other words, we have defied nature's most significant rule in keeping us healthy, which is separating the fiber from the carbohydrate.

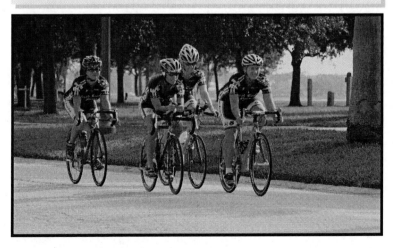

South Tampa girls going for a ride

Fiber Balances the Intestinal Tract

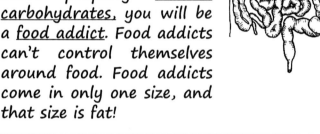

Fiber balances the intestinal tract with healthy chemicals that clean out the garbage. If you lack these important chemicals, your intestines become a toxic dump. This results in poor health and leads to obesity. If you don't properly <u>balance carbohydrates,</u> you will be a <u>food addict</u>. Food addicts can't control themselves around food. Food addicts come in only one size, and that size is fat!

Cave Men Weren't Stupid, They Did Not Process Food

The idea of separating carbohydrates from fibers is a new concept for the body, something man invented in the last few hundred years, which goes against everything nature would have us do. Processed foods are man's intervention of separating and removing fiber, (nature's package), and placing the carbohydrate in a man-made package. The problem is we can't eat man's package; it is usually cardboard with a colorful picture on it.

In fact, nature was so deliberate in maintaining a balance of fiber and carbohydrates that it designed foods with a higher percentage of carbohydrates to also have more fiber in them. Nature is so smart that it knew our bodies could not handle excessive amounts of carbohydrates without the assistance of fiber. For example, one cup of beans or grains is loaded with 40 grams of carbohydrates and 16 grams of fiber. Nature insured food that was loaded with starchy carbohydrates also needed fiber to insure slow steady absorption. In comparison, one cup of broccoli has less than 5 grams of carbohydrates so 4 grams of fiber is all that is needed. This is proof that nature knew exactly what it was doing to keep us healthy. The truth is that nature's intention for us is optimum health, and man's intention is keeping a few very rich. Need proof on man's motives? Check out one serving of cookies, chips, or white bread. Each has 40 grams of carbohydrates and less than 1 gram of fiber. So why do you get fooled and taken for a ride? Because the food industry is really good at making sure, *"You can't only eat just one,"* and you don't know why you can't. Now, you do, and now you won't be fooled again.

Nature's Design

	Carbs	Protein	Fiber
Beans	40	18	16
Brocolli	5	2	4

Man's Design

Cookies	40	0	0

"The balancing act that can save your life!"

Carbohydrate Balance

Most Americans are obsessed and fear-stricken with the starchy stuff inside the plant, the carbohydrate. This is the story of what happens once the carbohydrate is absorbed through the intestinal tract and enters the bloodstream. Keep in mind this is only one side of a two-sided story. It is a huge mistake to think it is just about carbohydrate balance. Total balance is when you know how both fiber and carbohydrates work together just like nature designed.

THE THREE FACTORS OF CARBOHYDRATE BALANCE

1. Using Carbohydrates for their **Designated Purpose**

2. The Correct **Amount & Proper Timing** of Carbohydrates

3. The **Sweet & Fat Survival Trait** in Our Genes

---

1. Using Carbohydrates for Their Designated Purpose

How it Works

Once carbohydrates enter the intestinal tract, they are separated from fiber, and at the same time, broken down into a simple sugar called glucose. It is only when they become glucose that they are ready to be absorbed into the bloodstream and delivered to all the cells. Unlike fiber that remains in the intestinal tract, a carbohydrate's job begins once it enters the bloodstream and is in circulation. Glucose is the juice cells use to operate. This sugar greatly affects the muscles and brain that depend on it to function. The problem is that the body can't wait until you figure out which foods are the best fuels. It has to keep you moving and the brain working 24 hours a day, seven days a week. Remember, the body doesn't have to keep you moving well or thinking clearly. It just has to keep you alive. In times of survival, or when carbs aren't available, the body has the ability to convert other foods besides carbohydrates into fuel. It does what it has to so that you can keep going.

Purpose Driven Life

A carbohydrates' designated purpose is to provide your body with fuel for energy. No other food has the capacity to do this with the same efficiency as carbohydrates. Carbohydrates want to live a purpose-driven life. A carbohydrate's sole purpose for existing, the reason why it is on this planet, is to provide your muscles and brain a clean, efficient, energy-producing fuel.

Protein and Fats Can be Forced to do the Job of a Carbohydrate

All food can be broken down into glucose. That includes protein, fat, and the excess fat you carry around. If you are eating food of any kind or even surviving off stored body fat, the metabolism ensures there is always glucose available for muscle and brain function. Although the body can make glucose from any food, the issue isn't glucose availability, but what happens to the metabolism in the process of getting the glucose. The cumbersome process the body has to go through to convert protein and fats into fuel causes a strain on the liver and kidneys, as well as causing dehydration, which leads to muscle fatigue, cramping, and mineral imbalance. It also creates a slightly acidic environment that makes you more susceptible to harm from bacteria and viruses.

Carbohydrates are the only foods that don't cause stress to the body during this conversion process. The body prefers to use the cleanest-burning fuel it can find, and that is exactly what carbohydrates are—clean, hassle-free fuels. There are no side effects. It is an easy conversion, because this is exactly what nature intended these foods to be used for.

The Carbohydrate Purpose

When you force the body to use less-efficient fuels, as when carbohydrates are restricted, and the body has no alternative but to break down protein and fat for energy fuels, there will always be an internal battle, because the body wants the fuels that are easier to convert and cleaner to use like carbohydrates. The stress and energy your body goes through to convert less efficient fuels into glucose, steals energy from you. It is hard to feel motivated and active when your muscles are sore and you have overall fatigue. This leads to less muscle growth and a higher percentage of body fat. It is what happens when carbs are **not** allowed to live their purpose-driven life inside of you.

---

2. The Correct Amount & Proper Timing of Carbohydrates Keep Balance.

There are two factors that determine the right number and proper timing of carbohydrates. One is the **immediate consumption** of a carbohydrate, and the other is the **reserve** of carbohydrates maintained in the body.

Nothing will cause more irritability and overall fatigue than getting the quantity and timing of carbohydrates wrong.
It causes a type of food addiction where the only foods that taste good are the ones you are trying to stay away from. This type of food addiction alters your palate where vegetables and fruits do not appeal to you.

Perhaps the only types of food that taste good are the high-carbohydrate, low-fiber ones. Healthy foods stop tasting good to you. In some cases, you lose an appetite for healthful food, or even food at all. Individuals with this addiction may not be overweight, but they still suffer from carbohydrate addiction, and they are harming their bodies.

Children and young adults fall victim to this type of addiction. They don't like vegetables, fruits, or any foods unless it is white pasta, white bread, chips, sweetened juices, candy, colas, fries, coffee, rich drinks, and any other foods rich in sugar and low in fiber. This type of diet results in imbalances of all kinds, and it creates a domino effect that leads to malnutrition, low-energy, and ultimately, weight gain.

The reason you have this addiction in the first place is that you have trained your body to want only carbohydrates by themselves, without protein or fiber. When carbohydrates are eaten this way, they enter the blood stream quickly and cause the body to release a surge of insulin. Insulin is the hormone responsible for delivering and storing sugar in the muscles and brain. It is a natural process, except when there is an overload of sugar. This excess sugar causes the body to release more insulin than normal.

Excess insulin caused from excess sugar puts your body in a chemical imbalance that results in craving more sugar, while becoming more efficient at storing fat.

What makes matters even worse is that most processed foods where the fiber has been removed also have more sugar added. This causes a huge spike in insulin. When insulin is surging in our body at higher levels than normal, it causes fatigue, mood swings, depression, and promotes fat storage. That's right, excess insulin surging through the blood encourages the body to become more efficient at storing fat. This high sugar spike triggers an increase in LDL (low-density lipoproteins). LDLs are the bad fats associated with heart disease and obesity.

High-sugar carbohydrates by themselves make you fatter and addicted to sugar. This puts you at risk for serious illnesses, such as Type II Diabetes, a condition where the cells become resistant to the constant surge of insulin and refuse to respond. It doesn't have to be a lot of sugar. Just one hard candy can cause a spike. Even healthy sugars like fruit juice can cause an insulin surge, all because an over-load of sugar was eaten with no fiber or protein to slow down the process. With this type of addiction, you may not eat large amounts of carbohydrates at one time with an uncontrollable urge to stop, but instead, you find you want to eat carbohydrates all day long. They are all you like to eat. In fact your body craves them.

Fiber and protein keep the carbohydrates in the intesti-nal tract longer which means carbohydrates are released into the bloodstream slower. This was nature's original de-sign, which means you have less insulin circulating in your blood.

Immediate carbohydrate consumption seems to be what every diet program focuses on, and is frequently referred to as the glycemic index or carb-free lifestyle. These diets are trying to save you from the insulin rush that happens when sugar is eaten in the wrong amounts at the wrong times. This alone is not the solution, because it is not the only fac-tor in balancing carbs. To focus only on the glycemic index or carb-free foods actually triggers another imbalance. This other carbohydrate imbalance is just as serious and preva-lent and not well known. I call it the **carbohydrate reserve factor**. That's just a fancy name I give for your body striving to keep a reserve of carbohydrates available for you to ac-cess, so you can move more freely and think clearly. If you eliminate or even restrict carbohydrates, the reserve will be-come depleted, thus signaling the body to tell the brain to eat more carbohydrates to replenish a low reserve.

Unfortunately, when reserves get too low, the body craves the wrong types of carbs. It is just hoping to get the quickest sugar it can get its hands on. The problem is that the brain doesn't think clearly once your reserve gets too low. This triggers irrational behavior, which leads to another type of addiction, and that is **binge eating**.

The real whammy is when both addictions occur simultaneously. Put simply, one addiction can cause the other to occur. Keeping the carb reserves too low promotes binging and out-of-control eating, which perpetuates the large amounts of carbs at one time. This keeps you trapped in a vicious cycle of abuse, where the only thing you want is what you shouldn't eat, and you can't stop eating foods that taste so good.

Bottom Line:

You have to learn how to balance your immediate carbohydrate consumption while maintaining your carbohydrate reserve. The six steps help you do this, and if you learn this process, carbohydrates will never give you a problem again. You will be able to walk away from foods you would have never been able to resist before. The more you can walk away, the more weight you will permanently lose.

Carbohydrate Reserve

The number of carbohydrates needed in your reserve is determined by your activity level. When carbohydrates are restricted for highly active people, the reserve can be depleted within one to two days. The body's ability to convert proteins and fats into fuel because of a lack of carbohydrates does not fix a low carbohydrate reserve problem. This type of low-carb reserve imbalance actually puts the body on red alert for *fiber less, bad-for-you*, carbohydrates. This means you will be a victim of uncontrollable urges for carbohydrate-rich foods such as sweets and chips—foods that your body prefers to convert easily and quickly to bring your reserve up to the level needed to support your activity.

As soon as your tongue tastes an indulgence of the carbohydrates you have been depriving yourself of, it is as if the brain shuts down, and you eat the entire bag, cake, loaf, or whatever is put in front of you. This is the body's way of getting back what you have deprived it. This is not something an intelligent person does but it is something that happens to intelligent people who have a food addiction. Get over the fact that it is you. It is the chemical state you put yourself in and you can fix it by knowing how to maintain carbohydrate balance.

Most people become obsessed and overwhelmed with the time and energy involved in maintaining a rigorous exercise schedule just so they can eat a few extra calories. They become scared to death of what they would become if they didn't exercise with such regularity and intensity. They will tell you it is easier to exercise obsessively then try and control their binging.

The same type of scenario happens when people get trapped into a Monday-Friday carb-restrictive diet plan so that they can treat themselves to the weekend of binging. They live for the weekends, only to find every Monday morning brings 5-8 pound weight gain with fatigue, bloating, and an enormous urge to repeat the cycle. Although some people are convinced this will work, they get caught in this vicious diet trap and eventually get fatter. They eat twice as much as they normally would on the weekends, and they are less motivated to move vigorously during the week.

This type of lifestyle promotes food addiction and creates an eating disorder. It makes you fatter, slows down your metabolism, and results in fatigue and depression. Although it is indeed a method some people use to control their weight, it is not a permanent solution, and eventually it catches up with them. Every year on this method, they get fatter.

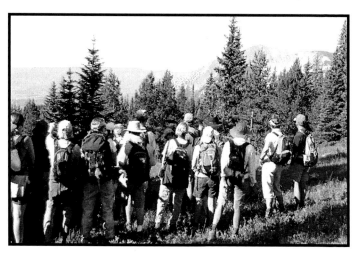

Only a few youngsters in this group of senior citizens embarking on a 12,000 ft. climb

Susan' restriction = addiction

Susan is an athlete who would tell you her sole purpose for her two- to three-hour gym workouts is to keep her from being obese. Although she only struggles with 10-15 pounds of extra weight, she swears she would weigh over 50 pounds more if not for her relentless gym regimen. Susan really watches what she eats during the day; breakfast and lunches are very healthy choices of vegetables proteins and a few fruits. Although Susan's diet is very healthy, and she seldom feels hungry, her activity level requires a large carbohydrate reserve. Her diet during the day doesn't support this high reserve level her workouts demand. She is so worried about gaining weight that most of her food choices are fat-free or reduced calories that are not properly balanced. This triggers insulin surges, causing her to fall into a deeper state of addiction. What is happening to Susan is she spends most of her day restricting carbohydrates only to struggle with a full-blown addiction every evening. She's in a vicious cycle of food addiction that makes her a slave to the gym to burn off the binge of the night before. This then perpetuates an eating disorder where the only amount of weight loss occurs when she increases her exercise.

How to fix Susan

If Susan balanced her carbs throughout the day, she wouldn't be in a depleted state in the evening hours. She would have more carbohydrates available during her activity, which means she would work harder, become more muscular, and have a leaner body. This also holds true for those people who use the weekends to make up for depleted reserves Monday through Friday, following the same pattern as Susan, but using a longer time period. There is enough evidence to prove this doesn't work. Susan and the other weekday worriers need to <u>balance their carbohydrate reserve</u>. Otherwise, they will eat five times more the number of calories in the evening than if they were balanced during the day.

The Right Amount of Carbohydrates Needed in Your Reserve

You have a choice. You can either manage your carbs, or they will manage you. If you allow your carb reserve to become depleted, you are putting your body in the driver's seat, and you can expect an out-of-control ride, one that results in fatigue and obesity. A better bet is to learn what it takes to maintain the carb reserve, so food will not control you. Hopefully, you have figured out that restricting carbohydrates just to drop a few pounds will eventually catch up with you. You will find your favorite delights irresistible because your reserve is depleted and your body is literally crying out for more and can't stop at one. This requires understanding your own personal carbohydrate range. Obviously you will require more carbohydrates the days you exercise than the days you don't.

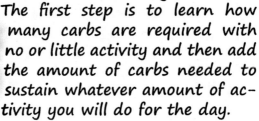

Carbs & Activity
The first step is to learn how many carbs are required with no or little activity and then add the amount of carbs needed to sustain whatever amount of activity you will do for the day.

If you consume your carbohydrates around your activity, then you get an added benefit of more energy during your activity. In other words, more energy when you need it increases your metabolism resulting in a leaner body.

How to Count Carbohydrates

All packaged carbohydrates, such as cereals, breads, crackers, pasta and beans, have a food label that will tell you the number of grams per serving. This will help you decide how many servings will help you reach your reserve. Be careful because you still need to consider the **immediate consumption** rule. Too much sugar at one time, with no fiber or protein, will cause an insulin surge that will put you in a tail spin, even if your reserves are at optimum levels.

Nutrition Facts

Serving Size 1/2 cup (about 82g)
Servings Per Container 8

Amount Per Serving

Calories 200   Calories from Fat 130

	% Daily Value*
Total Fat 14g	22%
Saturated Fat 9g	45%
Trans Fat 0g	
Cholesterol 55mg	18%
Sodium 40mg	2%
Total Carbohydrate 17g	6%
Dietary Fiber 1g	4%
Sugars 14g	
Protein 3g	

Vitamin A 10%	•	Vitamin C 0%
Calcium 10%	•	Iron 6%

*Percent Daily Values are based on a 2,000 calorie diet. Your daily values may be higher or lower depending on your calorie needs:

	Calories:	2,000	2,500
Total Fat	Less than	65g	80g
Saturated Fat	Less than	20g	25g
Cholesterol	Less than	300mg	300 mg
Sodium	Less than	2,400mg	2,400mg
Total Carbohydrate		300g	375g
Dietary Fiber		25g	30g

Calories per gram:
Fat 9 • Carbohydrate 4 • Protein 4

For the foods that don't have labels, such as produce, I have a rule-of-thumb calculation that works pretty well. If you want the exact amount, you can Google any food for nutrition information, and you will get several websites that can assist you.

Rule-of-Thumb – Carbohydrate Calculation for Foods That Don't Have Labels:

1 cup of fruit	20 grams Carbs
½ cup beans	20 grams Carbs
½ cup pasta	20 grams Carbs
1 slice bread	20 grams Carbs
1 small potato	20 grams Carbs
¼ cup nuts & seeds	10 grams Carbs
1 cup of vegetable	5 grams Carbs
Meat, chicken, fish	0 grams Carbs

What the Pro's Say About Your Daily Carbohydrate Reserve

The American Heart Association recommends that no one should have fewer than 80 grams per day of carbs. The diet examples they give include a healthy range of 180-250 grams per day, which works out to a daily percentage of 40-55 percent of total calories. The American Heart Association realizes it takes a lot more than 80 grams per day to be healthy and active, which is the key to being lean.

The government recommends a daily allowance of 45 to 65 percent of your caloric intake from carbs, which amounts to approximately 180-250 grams. (The Government's recommendation panel consists of qualified registered dieticians and physicians who are chosen from their peers and are the most respected in their field.) The government's experts recommend eating carbs from whole food sources, such as whole grains, beans, nuts, fruits, and vegetables, which means they're recommending that you eat carbohydrates and fiber together.

At least the experts in Washington understand nutrition and give solid recommendations, but unfortunately, they are powerless to do anything to persuade the food industry.

A registered dietician may recommend a program for weight loss that includes 40 to 55 percent of your total daily calories from carbs, which is approximately in the range of 800-1,000 calories, based on a 1,600 – 2,000 calorie day diet. Registered dieticians know all about carbohydrate balance, and their goal is to keep your carbohydrate reserves at optimal levels so you will have the fuel to move and think clearly, as well as engage in less addictive behavior.

Keep Carbohydrates at 180-250 Grams or 45-65 Percent of Total Daily Calories.

A good starting point for most people is in the range of 180-250 grams of carbohydrates per day. This is an approximate range that comes to 45- 65 percent of total daily calories for the average person who doesn't exercise. You have to experiment and get a feel for where you may be. Remember, your reserve can fluctuate. One way of knowing if you are keeping your range too low is if it feels as if it takes an enormous amount of self control just to stop at one chip or one cookie. If your reserves are maintained, you should be able to have just one bite or one cookie and feel satisfied. If your carbohydrate reserves are depleted, you will eat twice as many carbs as you would have if you had maintained your reserves. Keeping a box of Godiva chocolates close by helps me know if my reserves are balanced. Just like that naturally thin person we spoke about earlier, I can have one chocolate and feel satisfied.

Adding Exercise to Your Day Increases Your Reserve

Once you add exercise into your daily activity, you change the reserve equation. Depending on the amount and intensity of exercise, your carbohydrates reserve may need an extra 60-200 grams!

For Every Hour of Exercise, Add 40-60 Grams of Carbs

This means the days you don't exercise, you may need 180-250 grams of carbs, and the days when you do, it is more in the range of 250-400 grams.

Keep Your Carbohydrate Reserve at the Right Level

This is an example of what 50 percent of an average day's worth of carbs would look like to maintain balanced reserves. Assume a daily caloric value of 2,000 calories.

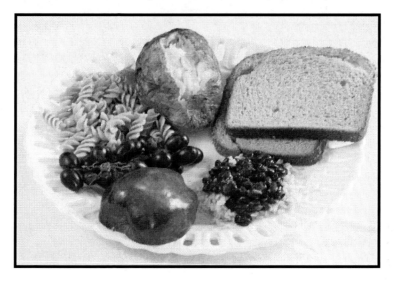

This doesn't include protein or fat daily requirements. This illustrates how many carbohydrates are needed through out the day to maintain a healthy carb reserve **without exercise.**

Food	Calories	Carb (Grams)
2 slices whole grain bread	200	38
1 cup whole grain pasta	200	48
2 fruits	150	40
1cup beans	210	40
½ cup rice	110	20
1 baked potato – medium	200	45
Total	**1070**	**211**

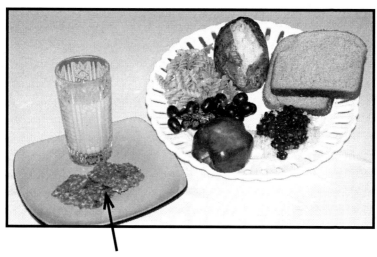

Add approx 50 grams of carbs for every one hour of exercise

Illustration shows 90 grams of carbs are added with 90 minutes to two hours of exercise.

Food	Calories	Carb (grams)
2 slices whole grain bread	200	36
1 cup whole grain pasta	200	45
2 fruits	150	40
1 cup beans	210	40
1/2 cup rice	110	20
1 baked potato	200	45
Add: 90 minutes of exercise		
Energy bar	350	45
1 cup juice	150	45
Total	**1,580**	**316**

*This doesn't include the daily requirement of proteins and fats.

Competitive athletes (and our friend Susan we spoke of earlier), could easily require an additional 90-200 grams for 2-3 hours of exercise, for a total requirement of 300-350 grams per day!

Fuel Your Workout

Ideally, if you can eat these extra carbohydrates around your activity, and not late at night as a binge, you will get an added benefit of an awesome workout that gives you awesome results.

Everyone's range can be slightly different and can fluctuate daily. Two factors that influence your range are the amount of muscle you carry around, and the amount of muscle you use, which as I explained, is determined by your activity level. The higher percentage of muscle to fat requires more calories to maintain, and since muscles feed off of carbohydrates for fuel, this could mean your carbohydrate reserve could be 30-40 grams more, just because you are more muscular. That is correct! You can increase your metabolism just because you have more muscles. Clinically obese individuals will have much lower carbohydrate reserves to maintain, but with an exercise program, this will change for them as well.

Soon we will work together to estimate your reserve based on the life you want to live. For now, keep going.

Carbohydrate Reserve Summary

To maintain an adequate reserve of carbohydrates, the range will fall between 180-250 grams per day for the average person. This is approximately half the caloric intake of carbohydrates, assuming an average intake of 1,800-2,000 calories per day. The carbohydrates should be evenly spread throughout the day. It is best if carbs are centered around any activity to enhance performance.

If sugar-processed carbohydrates are used to satisfy your carb reserve, you risk insulin addiction problems that will eventually be the only foods you want and you can't understand why.

Why experts recommend low-carb diets.

In some cases low-carb diets are recommended for a very brief period, maybe two-to-three weeks, to kick-start a weight-loss program. This is done more as a confidence booster. People have more motivation when they see immediate results. If these professionals have your best interests in mind, they should be telling you that the program that keeps it off permanently is very different from the quick weight-loss program they have you on.

Weight-loss centers focus on the weight and not the life of the person. Most people are fooled into believing that once they are thin, they can magically figure out the program required for staying thin. Let's face it. There is a lot of money in weight loss. Most professionals assume once you are thin, you will know how to stay thin. Their job is to get the weight off, not balance your life. Unless you know how to balance your diet, you will always be trying to lose weight.

The truth is that quick weight-loss programs that get you thin are not the same programs that keep you there. Why not just figure out the program that keeps you there and try and live that? That is what this book is about, and the only real program that works.

Barb is one baked potato away from an addiction.

When Barb participated in her first six-step workshop, she decided diets were a thing of the past, and she was dedicated to learning the process and then applying it to her life. I never ask people what they weigh, but I would guess that she carried what looked like an extra 50 pounds. Although she dropped only seven pounds, she went from a size 14 to a size 4.. Barb gained muscle, which weighs three times more than fat. She was working hard all year, not realizing as her body and activity levels were changing, so were her carbohydrate requirements. Barb's reserves changed dramatically after the first year, but so had Barb's body. One day in the grocery store her 10-year-old son stopped her from having an addiction meltdown. Barb's reserves were depleted, and she was on a ravaging hunt, loading her cart with foods she felt compelled to buy. After hearing his mother explain the six-step process, her son told her that she was only one baked potato away from thousands of calories of total destruction. Barb went home, had a baked potato and was saved. Barb realized that 200 grams of carbohydrates per day wasn't enough to sustain her muscular, active body. She increased her daily requirement to 250 grams, which is one more baked potato per day. Now, when she rides her bike, she takes an energy bar with her.

3. The Sweet & Fat Survival Trait
in Our Genes

When our <u>Genes</u> Aren't Working With our <u>Jeans</u>

It isn't at all difficult to understand why over 65 percent of us are fat, and by the year 2020, it is predicted that over 88 percent of us will be overweight. Let's face it. You live in a hostile food environment that is more about corporate gain than your health, and the only way you're going to save yourself from being a statistic is to be smart. Unfortunately, just when you think your intelligence and due-diligence is working for you, there is one more nail that could seal your coffin. This last factor in carbohydrate balance has to do more with something you can't control, but if you work on the six step process it shouldn't be a major concern. It is worth mentioning because it can explain a lot of irrational behavior.

What I'm referring to is a **human trait that is built into our DNA.** It has been there for millions of years for the sole purpose of helping us make good food choices. Nature didn't provide an instruction book on the best food to eat, but instead etched it into our DNA. Nature had to make sure we would eat foods that were the healthiest.

This was accomplished by making healthy foods sweet and fat, and then making our bodies desire those foods. That is really meaningful if you are a caveman roaming the forest and need to depend on a gut feeling. This human trait makes it almost impossible to stay away from sweet and fatty foods.

Sweets and Fats in Nature

Foods in nature taste the sweetest when they are the ripest. This is when they have soaked up the highest nutritive value from the vine or tree. In the old days, animals that were fat were the healthiest game, and the ones we preferred to hunt, because these animals tasted the best. Foods in nature that are at their peak for nutritional value will be sweet and fat, and our body loves to eat them. In fact, your body will tell you it is your best choice, even if it's not.

This perfect system nature designed would have worked great even a century ago, but in the world we live in today, it is a disaster. Since the last 100 years, we now live in a food environment in which the sweetest and fattest foods are the unhealthiest. Unfortunately, we have a trait from the good old days that doesn't recognize the current reality. The DNA instructions that kept us alive for the last million years are slowly killing us today.

This trait makes carbohydrate addiction really difficult to control. It sounds crazy, like something out of a horror flick. But this special trait built into our DNA makes us instinctively go for the sweetest and fattest foods, even if they are the worse choice. Combine this with food addiction, and it would be short of a miracle if you aren't overweight. No wonder so many of us struggle.

It is no accident that food manufacturers know we will always pick the sweetest and fattest foods. We don't even need to taste the food. It just needs to be sweet and fat. The ultimate trickery has just occurred, because the body believes it is choosing the food that is the best for us, while these very foods are the worse.

High fructose corn syrup may be the highest deception of all! High fructose corn syrup is a manufactured food, one that is produced in a laboratory that has 1.7 times the sweetness of anything natural.

Imagine a young child or even an adult confronted with a piece of cake or an apple. Your body tells you to choose the cake, even though your mind is fully aware that the apple is a better choice. Still, it is the cake you want. All right, now think of this trait combined with a food addiction, and the challenge is even greater.

You will never be able to remove the sweet and fat trait from your DNA, nor can you fault the food industry for trying to make a buck. They are giving us exactly what we desire, and we are the ones buying their products. The only defense you have is to understand what is happening and keep your body balanced. When your body is balanced, food addictions do not control you. Even if you have been programmed to eat the sweetest and fattest, you won't be **dying** to have it. You will be able to step back and reason with your body, and you won't be in a chemical state of irrational behavior.

I hope you now have a better understanding that this has very little to do with willpower! It is truly a chemical addiction you have the power to change.

The Fact You are Fat Has Nothing to do With Your Emotional Baggage

I get so tired of listening to trainers tell their clients that their emotional state of affairs is limiting their body to lose weight. Why can't they just admit diets don't work, especially the one they put their clients on. Instead, when their client gains the weight back the trainer gets paid again, the process starts over, and the client is given the diet bible. The clients never blame the trainer. In fact, they are convinced the reason they failed is because they couldn't stay on the program. They lacked self control, let themselves slip back, fell off the wagon, you name it. And then they hire the same trainer!

Since the trainer plans on using the exact same program, maybe the "improved version," to get the exact same results, they have to find an alibi. Here is the old time favorite: *"My client has emotional baggage, and she depends on comfort food to eat her way out of her problems"*

It amazes me that intelligent people fall for this bull! Everyone has emotional baggage, but not everyone is controlled by food. I'm not saying that some trainers don't have solid exercise and diet programs, just be realistic in the fact they make money when you're dependant on them and their program.

What's Behind the Diet Program You Are On?

It's not carbohydrates that make us fat, but our inability to balance them. Fiber plays a significant role in this process.

Diets ask you to follow a road map, which can sometimes be good, but can also be a disaster. I'm not saying road maps aren't good or even necessary. I'm just suggesting to get a better understanding of what's behind the diet program you may have decided to follow.

Take Back What is Yours!

Stop believing that it is only about weight loss, and start believing it is all about finding the most optimum plan. Diet is a word that is being used by an industry trying to make money on your unstable condition. Start believing you have the ultimate control. Take back what is yours.

SEVEN

FIBER

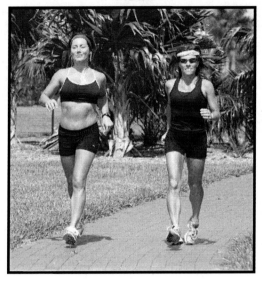

Removing Fiber is a Bad Idea

If you have hung around this far, I'm sure you're well informed that removing the fiber from a carbohydrate is a really bad idea. It makes you fat, and increases your risk for certain illnesses. Research supports this with their claim that a **high consumption of fiber is the single most important factor in the fight against obesity and the prevention of diseases.** Fiber has a lot of health benefits that work with carbohydrates in keeping you balanced. It is well worth understanding why and how this magical substance could save you a lot of money in doctor bills, and possibly save your life!

As we mentioned before, fiber is what holds the seeds, stems, and leaves together. It doesn't break down into a simple sugar or get sifted away like its partner, the carbohydrate. Instead, fiber remains in the intestinal tract providing your body with a host of chemicals that are responsible for many functions such as: cleaning your body of toxic waste, providing balance for the colony of intestinal bacteria, creating healthy fatty acids that aid in weight loss, keeping insulin levels steady, and making you feel full with no calories.

Fiber happens to be where most of nature's cancer-fighting nutrients are stored. Fiber cannot only save your life, but empower you to never have to diet again. Fiber, more than any other food on the planet, can prevent disease and control obesity. No wonder it has been referred to as the "magic bullet" in the control of obesity and overall health.

Americans consume less than one-fourth the recommended daily allowance of fiber, which could explain why obesity is a national epidemic, and our health care system is burdened with more than 70 percent of all diseases that could have been prevented just by simply understanding good health. Not to mention that most people can't afford to get sick.

THE TWO BENEFITS OF FIBER BALANCE:

1. **Fiber cleans the body of toxic chemicals.**

2. **Fiber contains materials that are significant in the prevention of most diseases.**

1. Fiber Cleans our Body of Toxic Chemicals

Fiber uses two methods of removing toxic material from the digestive tract. One is through a fiber called **soluble,** and the other through a fiber called **insoluble.** All plant foods have a certain proportion of these two types of fiber. These remarkable cleaning agents become activated once they are in our digestive tract.

Soluble fibers break down into a sludgy material. This sludgy material serves as a filter that removes toxic chemicals from the foods that travel through the digestive tract. This sludgy, gooey material coats the insides of the intestinal tract. It has an affinity for toxins and bad fats, such as the LDL fat, which is found in bad cholesterol and is a precursor to heart disease. Toxins get trapped in this gooey material and are not allowed to be absorbed into the bloodstream. These bad fats stick to the gel and are washed out of the body.

Soluble fiber pulls and traps bad fat and toxins in your digestive tract, then removes them from the body.

Soluble fibers are found in plant foods that have gum or *pectin,* which are gel-forming textures that break down into a gooey sludge once in the intestinal tract. The fiber foods that have a higher proportion of soluble fibers are: oats, legumes, barley, apples, citrus fruits, strawberries, soy, rice, potatoes and carrots.

Insoluble fibers also remain in the intestinal tract, but instead of breaking down into a gooey material, they remain more intact and are broken down into small plant particles. These small particles act as tiny scrub brushes that scrape the intestinal wall, removing toxic waste that gets lodged in the crevices.

Insoluble fiber act as tiny scrub brushes cleaning the insides of our intestines removing toxins that stick to the walls.

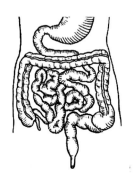

Keep in mind the intestinal tract is approximately 25 feet of tubing that fits into the size of a small grapefruit under the stomach. There are plenty of hairpin turns where waste material can sit and ferment. The longer this material is allowed to sit in the intestines, the higher risk of developing certain cancers, as well as the possibility of toxins being re-absorbed back into the bloodstream. The highest sources of insoluble fibers are found in wheat bran, whole grains, vegetables, fruits, and seeds.

Why a Fiber Pill or Powder Doesn't Do the Same Job

Fiber tablets, pills or powders, the commercial grades of fiber supplements, help move material through the intestinal tract, but don't have the same balancing benefit. Although it is better than allowing material to sit in the intestinal tract for days, it does not have the same health benefit as eating the foods that are rich in soluble and insoluble fibers found naturally in plants. The reason is that natural fibers also have chemicals that provide metabolic benefits, and serve as prevention for cancers and other diseases. Fiber that is processed, the kind you find in commercial fiber supplements, lacks these powerful chemicals. In other words, they help clean your intestinal tract, similar to the way a laxative does, but you are missing out on all the other metabolic benefits fiber has to offer.

2. Fiber Contains Materials That are Significant in the Prevention of Most Diseases.

Fiber Helps With Weight Loss.

Fiber stays in the stomach longer, which makes you feel full as well as satisfied. Fiber allows you to eat more food with fewer calories. When this happens, you eat less and more slowly. When you're full on fewer calories, eventually you'll weigh less.

Fiber Controls Blood Sugar

Fiber slows the rate at which food is absorbed into the bloodstream. When food is slowly absorbed into the blood, the hormone *insulin* is also released more slowly. This means your blood sugar is more stable. In the case of white flour and white sugar, there is very little fiber or protein to slow down digestion. Insulin is released in excess and quickly. At first you feel a sugar rush, but within an hour, you're fatigued and irritable. Choosing a high-fiber protein choice like oatmeal controls your mood and lessens fat promotion unlike a high-sugar, low-fiber choice such as a cupcake or danish that causes food addiction with a propensity to gain weight through an increase in body fat.

High Fiber Diets Decrease the Risk of Cancer

Colon and other cancers occur less frequently in societies that consume high-fiber diets. Fiber moves material through the intestines allowing less time for feces to build up in the colon. Waste that is allowed to sit in the intestinal tract may cause cancerous growth in the cracks and crevasses of the intestinal wall.

Fiber binds and removes these toxic materials, called *carcinogens*, from being absorbed into the bloodstream, as well as leaving beneficial bacteria in the lining of the intestinal wall that protects against harmful bacteria.

Fiber Promotes Healthy Bacteria in intestinal Lining

Our intestinal tract uses bacteria organisms to break down food, absorb nutrients, and make metabolic enzymes and proteins that are used to keep your immune system and all other systems running smoothly. The good bacteria, which are called **probiotics,** destroy harmful bacteria, which is why you want a lot of them. They are your first line of defense in the war on germs. If you have low numbers of good bacteria, which happens with a low-fiber diet, the bad bacteria is allowed to multiply.

You can never rid yourself of bad bacteria; you can only stop them from growing and making you sick. The perfect recipe for bad bacteria overload is a diet high in processed foods and low in fiber, such as white flour and sugar foods. Excess sugar and low fiber create just the kind of environment that bad bacteria thrive on. Keeping the colony of good bacteria alive and large in numbers may be the only natural defense you have. It is your first line of defense in the fight against harmful substances.

In simple language, good bacteria need fiber in the intestinal tract to perform all the jobs that are necessary to maintain your health.

The soluble and insoluble fibers we discussed earlier are commonly referred to as **prebiotics.** These fiber materials create the perfect condition for the good bacteria to flourish and perform the tasks they were designed to do. Good bacteria needs the materials found in fiber for fermentation, which is what keeps the intestinal tract balanced. Through this fermentation process, raw materials are formed that create a catalyst for other very important biological functions such as, inhibiting cholesterol synthesis, as well as enhance the absorption and retention of minerals such as calcium, magnesium, zinc and iron.

Good Bacteria Depend on Fiber to Function.

What a lot of people don't realize is that the maintenance of the good bacteria (probiotics) is a delicate balance that can be destroyed by poor food choices, stress, medications, pollutants, and age. When good bacteria are inadequate, the intestinal balance is in jeopardy. This gives the bad bacteria a great opportunity for a hostile takeover, which leaves you in a real mess. You won't know your intestinal tract is not balanced. There will be no indication of poor absorption and digestion of important nutrients. What happens is that you're eating, but your body isn't receiving. Obviously, this will make a difference in how you feel, and eventually, how you look.

Your intestinal tract is where it all begins. If it isn't functioning optimally, how can you expect to be energetic and getting the most out of the foods you eat? Studies show that eating this way can cause weight gain, fatigue, and uncomfortable medical symptoms you may never associate with poor intestinal imbalance.

Research indicates that irritable bowel syndrome, which affects 20 percent of the population, may be due to an over-growth of bad bacteria in the intestines. Over 80 percent of IBS cases had harmful bacteria over-growth in the intestinal tract. IBS symptoms range from, bloating, gas, abdominal pain, and constipation, to diarrhea. Most physicians do not recognize IBS as an intestinal tract imbalance, and most people spend years suffering from a condition for which they are told there is no cure. Diets high in processed sugars and low in fiber contribute to this over-growth of harmful bacteria, which feeds on sugar and lives best in an environment of low fiber.

Ideally, you want to create a hostile environment for these harmful bacteria by keeping your intestines balanced and clean! That is exactly what soluble and insoluble plant fiber from fruits, vegetables, beans, and grains will do for you.

Antibiotics Kill the Good and Bad Bacteria

Although antibiotics kill harmful bacteria, they also kill the good bacteria. If you have been on antibiotics, it is important to eat foods that contain cultures of good bacteria (probiotics). Probiotics foods are found in fermented products such as yogurt (Activa yogurt) and Kumbucha, a fermented tea (synergy teas found in the refrigerated section of most health stores). These products contain helpful probiotic bacteria called lactobacillus and bifidobacteria. It can take several weeks of daily probiotics before your body is able to replenish itself after a bout of medicated antibiotic wipe-out. A good safe measure would be to try and include them in your diet on a regular basis.

Fiber Foods Contain Cancer-Fighting Properties

Plants are the only living organisms that are able to pull energy from the sun through a process called *photosynthesis* and soak up essential minerals from the soil. This makes plants unique from any other foods. The sun and earth energy is converted into chemicals that are stored in the leaves, stems, fruit, and seeds of the plant. This sun and earth energy produces phyto-chemicals which have the highest value for disease prevention of any foods on the planet.

I suppose if humans could eat dirt and lick sunlight, plants wouldn't need to do it for them. Since that is not the case, plants need to be an important part of our diets. More than 6,000 natural chemicals found in plants are part of this earth-energy phenomenon and they're showing promise in the prevention of certain cancers. It is the bright rich colors in vegetables, such as fruits, seeds, beans, and nuts show that highly nutritional chemicals exist in these plants. Think of the red in tomatoes and apple skins, the rich greens in kale and spinach, the bright orange in carrots and sweet potatoes.

Worthless Soil Equals Worthless Plants.

Plants need time to soak up the earth's energy. When they are picked green and not allowed to ripen on the vine, the plant has less time to soak up all the nutrients as nature intended. This means we get a less nutritious food.

Good soil is also critical. As we mentioned earlier, the plant's purpose is to pull minerals from the soil. A few minerals you may recognize are selenium, zinc, iron, and calcium. Farmers rotate their fields, so that the soil has time to rest and build back up the minerals that were soaked into the previously harvested crops.

Due to high-grade fertilizers, farmers today are not as dependant on field rotation as they were in the past. These advancements allow plants to grow on low quality soil. Some plants can grow in Styrofoam if given enough fertilizer. Although the plant can look perfectly normal, and the fiber content seems to remain the same regardless of the poor growing conditions, the vitamins, minerals, and phyto-chemicals are affected. In other words, if you grow a plant on worthless soil, you get a worthless plant that can look and taste perfectly normal.

In other words, a plant grown on quality soil and allowed to ripen on the vine has double the nutritional quality than the plant that was picked green or grown in poor quality soil.

Research shows that the nutritional quality in plants can be reduced by over half when they are grown in poor quality soil.

Processed Food Kills Beneficial Chemicals

Once foods have been processed, as is the case with white flour, white breads, cookies, cakes, white pastas, white rice, chips, and most packaged shelf foods, the natural chemicals have been destroyed or removed. What usually remains is the starchy material minus the fiber and health benefits that were in the plant in its original form.

Being Popular isn't Always a Good Thing.

Processing has become popular in this country because it creates a long shelf life and sweeter food. Hopefully, at this point you are fully aware that when food tastes sweeter, we buy and eat more of it. The addictive nature of processed foods causes us to consume massive quantities of calorie-rich, poor-quality food. This has resulted in an obesity epidemic with out-of-control health care problems, because the only hope we had of health prevention was stripped from our foods and loaded with sugar to ensure we would become addicts to addictive substances similar to crack cocaine, but legal.

If the Government Requires Foods to be Fortified, Should We Worry?

About 70 years ago, when packaged food was really starting to take off, the government realized the removal of vitamins and minerals from our foods would create an epidemic of malnutrition. That is when the government required the food industry to fortify foods with vitamins and minerals. The sad truth is just a few vitamins and minerals were replaced, nothing in comparison to what the plant originally had. To make it worse, most people believe as long as it says, *"Fortified with vitamins and minerals,"* it is a higher quality food! WRONG! What you get is lower quality food that is advertised as being better for you and charged double for. I hope this sheds new light on packaging claims such as *"fortified"* or *"added nutrition."*

The Body Keeps a Balance of Acid and Alkaline

Another type of balance the body maintains is the level of acidity in our blood. We have built-in mechanisms that buffer us from ever becoming too acidic, or the other end of the scale, of being too alkaline. Either condition, in an extreme case, can cause death. Not to worry because the blood maintains a certain balance of acidity and alkalinity, and it does a really good job of keeping you out of a life-or-death situation. But just because you aren't dying doesn't mean you won't have a poor quality of life.

The lifestyle you choose can have a daily effect on the acid or alkaline balance. It is a very slight change in our internal environment, not a major fluctuation causing severe complications. But it is still enough of a change that it can cause poor health.

Research shows that even a very slight swing, a value that is tolerable for the body, not life threatening, can affect your health. All foods create a slight acidic or alkaline environment when we eat them. It has nothing to do with the sour taste found in foods such as what you taste in grapefruits, oranges and lemons. It has more to do with how these foods react once they hit your digestive tract.

Acidic and alkaline balance isn't just isolated to the foods we eat. Stress, pollution, medications, and even negative, anxiety-filled thoughts can cause a slightly acidic environment, not enough to cause a major shut-down, but enough to change your internal chemistry, resulting in a less optimal quality of life.

Research Indicates That Slight Acidity in the Blood is Affiliated with Certain Diseases.

Foods that create an acidic environment are the same ones that cause microscopic inflammation that have been linked to heart disease, arthritis, degenerative diseases, and premature aging. Microscopic inflammation isn't something you see or feel, but it secretly does damage to your cells. Acidity doesn't just promote inflammation. Research shows that bacteria and viruses love acidic environments also. This means you are more vulnerable to contracting colds and other illnesses when you create acidity.

A diet that consists of low-fiber, processed foods that are high in sugar and hydrogenated fats creates an acidic chemistry, which is a perfect environment for bad bacteria, inflammation, and obesity. These include foods such as white flour and sugar products, including cookies, chips, and high-sugar snack foods. Along with highly processed foods, animal foods that have no fiber, including meat, eggs, and cheese, when eaten in excess, create an acidic environment.

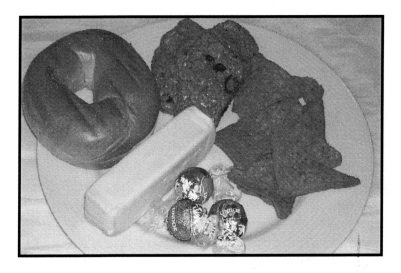

Animal foods, processed foods and sugary foods cause aciidity

Some diets promote an acidic state of ketosis as being a kick start for losing weight. Wrong! Ketosis is a metabolic process that happens when our body is forced into using proteins and fats for fuel, which is the case with a carbohydrate restrictive diet. This acidic imbalance dehydrates our cells and the resulting loss of water weight, combined with the high proteins, creates a metabolic imbalance that results in acidic internal body chemistry. This is very slight and tolerable, and many doctors do not view ketosis as being life threatening. Perhaps not short-term, but long-term it leads to serious illness.

For instance, diets high in animal proteins and processed foods cause acidity and also may result in *osteoporosis*, a fancy name given to bone loss. Imagine your skeletal structure melting away. It doesn't really melt, it just seems that way when the structure that holds you in place begins to disappear. The bones are brittle, and full of hollow holes. It is not a pretty sight when you are humped over, and the pain can be unbearable as your spinal cord disintegrates. This is what happens when you allow your body to pull calcium from your bones to balance the high levels of phosphorous contained in a highly acidic-high protein animal diet.

The point here is how one imbalance causes a cascade of others. A highly acidic internal chemistry is intertwined with carbohydrate addiction and linked to the improper use of proteins, which in turn causes bone loss, inflammation, fatigue, depression, and is associated with irritable bowel syndrome and an increase in infections. All of this leads to weight gain which happens to be a major risk factor for all diseases! What should be really disturbing is that doctors give clean bills of health while people are actually toxic dumps with all kinds of imbalances that manifest later into full-blown diseases.

> *Research shows that certain foods can boost your immunity by slightly changing the ph in the blood to more alkaline than acidic.*

There are not enough resources spent on prevention. After all, this is where it all starts and is still affordable. Preventing illness has everything to do with balance.

Alkaline Balance

There are certain plant foods that create a slight alkaline ph in the blood. Green, leafy vegetable are at the top of the list. The chlorophyll that gives these foods their green color has shown to have other remarkable properties besides just supplying us with essential vitamins, minerals, and phyto-chemicals.

These foods create a slightly different chemical environment in our body that happens to make you a poor host for bad bacteria and viruses. Every day you come in contact with potentially harmful substances. The best defense is to create a body where theses harmful agents don't want to stay and raise a family. The type of diet that keeps your body slightly alkaline is also the same one that is high in fiber from eating plants in their original form. The highest value foods are your colorful vegetables such as, squash, kale, spinach, broccoli, and zucchini, just to name a few.

Negative Thoughts Can Change Your Internal Chemistry

Food is not the only element that can affect your internal chemistry. Negative thoughts that cause you to become anxious, depressed, feelings of hopelessness and overwhelming stress of not being able to control your personal situation can affect your internal balance. Your thoughts can spark your body into wellness or illness.

What happens is that hormones release chemicals because of your thoughts. These hormones become the catalyst for other imbalances to occur. Research supports the high association between people under emotional stress and illness. When the chemicals produced from stress are allowed to circulate continually in excessive amounts, you set the stage for serious fall-out. This is all from the thoughts that your brain creates, and your brain can remove.

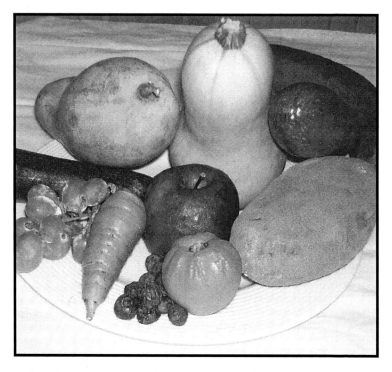

Colorful vegetables and whole unprocessed food promote alkalinity

Promotes an Acidic Environment	Promotes an Alkaline Environment
All animal food such as: dairy, meat, chicken, pork , bacon, butter.	Green leafy vegetables are the best.
Processed foods such as; hydrogenated fats, white flour, white sugar, and fried foods.	All other vegetables such as; zucchini, squash, broccoli, fruits such as: oranges, lemons, grapefruits, apples, bananas and other high fiber foods such as: beans, seeds nuts and to a lesser extent natural whole grains.
Negative thoughts, stress, depression and anxiety.	Laughter, meditation, prayer, happy mood and thoughts.

Daily Requirement

The recommended daily requirement of fiber is 25-40 grams per day. On average, most Americans consume less than 8 grams per day. There should be an equal mix of soluble and insoluble fibers, which is stated in the My pyramid information distributed by the government dietary council. It recommends; 3-5, ½ cup servings vegetables, 2-4 servings of fruit, 6-11 servings of grains(1 slice of bread or 1/2 cup cereal or pasta is an average serving) and or 2-3, ½ cup servings of beans or 2-3 ¼ serving nuts and seeds. Beans and grains will vary based on your carbohydrate requirement, which is determined by your activity as covered in the carbohydrate section. It looks like a lot of food, but it really isn't. When fiber remains in food, it takes up a lot of space, but doesn't cost you any calories. Just to prove my point, I calculated the daily fiber requirement based on the food pyramid requirements from the government . A healthy typical day of fiber can range anywhere from 25 grams to 60 grams.

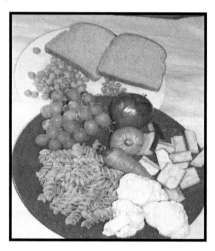

Typical Day of Fiber	Calories	Fiber
5 - ½ cup servings vegetables	150	10
2 fruits	160	6
1 cup beans	200	16
¼ cup nuts	160	3
2 slices whole wheat bread	160	4
1 cup whole wheat pasta	210	8
Total	**1040**	**47**

Now compare the typical American diet, which is loaded with white sugar and white flour alternatives.

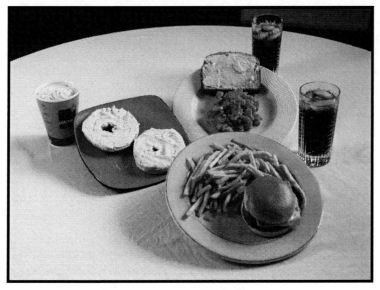

The typical American diet has twice the calories, with less volume of food, half the fiber and nutriients, with no probiotic health which results in more hunger, obesity and addiction.

Typical American Fiber	Calories	Fiber
Bagel with cream cheese	350	2
1 - 8 oz sweet coffee drink	300	0
2 colas	400	0
French fries - 2 servings	500	2
1 small chicken sandwich	350	2
1 cup macaroni and cheese	450	1
1 slice bread with butter	150	1
Total	**2,500**	**8**

If you compare the volume of food for each example, there is a big difference between 8 grams versus 42 grams of fiber. The first example has double the volume of food and nutrients with less than half the calories. In other words you get to eat twice as much food for half the calories, feel more full, and get healthier in the process, which research claims is a significant factor in losing weight.

In example two, you eat double the calories with half the nutrients, on less food which leads to poor health, low energy, food addiction and obesity, and what is really crazy is that you still feel hungry for more food.

Is Too Much Fiber Bad?

Just like everything, fiber needs to be eaten in moderation with your diet. Excessive amounts of anything, even if it is healthy, can create an imbalance and make you suddenly unhealthy. Although fiber is good for you, too much can be bad. Fiber in excess can cause a depletion of certain vitamins and minerals, and can bind other nutrients together that inhibit their absorption. You should not have watery stools, or intestinal cramping.

If you have lived most your life consuming 6-8 grams of fiber, you can not suddenly jump to 40 grams in one day. You have to give your body time to adjust, and your intestinal tract time to build up good bacteria. You will also have to increase your water intake. Fiber requires water to properly function once in the intestinal tract. I have had many clients tell me that they doubled their water intake once their fiber reached 30-35 grams after living on 6-8 grams per day most their life. It can take 1-2 months to adjust to the increase, and not everyone has enzymes that work perfectly with all fibers, which is necessary when breaking down fibers in the gut. This will require some experimentation in figuring out which fibers work best for you.

Counting Fiber:

Rule of Thumb Calculation for Foods that Don't Have Labels:

1 cup of fruit	4 grams of fiber
1 cup of vegetable	4 grams of fiber
½ cup beans	8 grams of fiber
¼ cup nuts and seeds	3 grams fiber
Meat, chicken fish	0 grams of fiber

The health benefit of fiber is a major factor in the health of our body. The daily requirement of 25-40 grams of fiber per day can significantly change your body chemistry to lower your risk for certain cancers, obesity and intestinal balance, enhancing your immunity and quality of life. Removing fiber from carbohydrates creates imbalances that cause inflammation, obesity and is associated with many cancers and illnesses.

Water, protein, carbohydrates and fiber all have their own rules for proper balance. Essential fats are no different. Certain fats will kill you, and other fats are critical for survival. Not knowing which ones do what may be life threatening. The next chapter will enlighten you.

EIGHT

CAN'T LIVE WITHOUT ESSENTIAL FATS

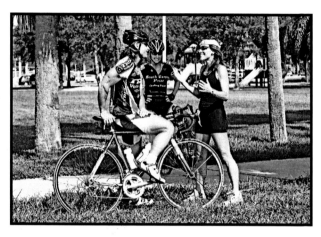

Much easier to keep up with this guy off the bike!

Essential Fats Are Important

Essential fats are so important that without them, we get sick. The problem is that most of the time we have no clue that this absence is what is making us sick. Physicians overlook that an essential fatty acid imbalance could be the cause of ailments such as dry, itchy skin, brittle hair and nails, digestion problems, irritable bowels, constipation, joint and muscle pain, poor concentration and depression. The truth is that essential fatty acid imbalances are responsible for health problems ranging from cardiovascular disease, digestive and stomach disorders, immune and nervous system dysfunctions, hormonal imbalances, and behavior and brain disorders.

What should really scare you is that essential fats are at dangerously low levels in the American diet and are only available through the food we eat, which means our bodies can't produce them. This means that if your diet lacks these essential fats, you are in big trouble. The research is overwhelming regarding how balancing these fats plays a significant role in how the body regulates itself. I believe this information could save your life and thousands of dollars in medical bills.

What Makes Essential Fats So Important?

These essential fats come from our food source and you will learn which foods have them and how to keep them balanced. I thought it was best to first explain the role these essential fats play in keeping us healthy. Although these essential fats serve many functions, the two major functions that stand out the most, and truly define their roles best, are what they do for our cells and hormones and how they regulate them.

Cellular Function

These fats have a huge effect on cellular membranes. Cell membranes are the outside layers of cells. The cell membrane determines what is allowed in and out of the cell, which is why it is very important to keep these membranes healthy. Essential fatty acids make cellular membranes flexible, more pliable. If they are stiff and rigid, they will be more prone to fractures and cracks that damage the cell wall and can ultimately damage what is inside. Keep in mind if the cell membrane is weak, the cell can't protect itself from invaders.

When these cells become rigid, they also lose their ability to hold water and other nutrients, which affects their ability to communicate with other cells. When cells can't communicate with other cells and lose their ability to protect themselves, the whole system becomes vulnerable. Once invaders are allowed inside cells, the DNA of the cell can get damaged. The DNA is where the cell gets its instructions. When this is impaired, the cell cannot function in the way that it was designed, resulting in poor health.

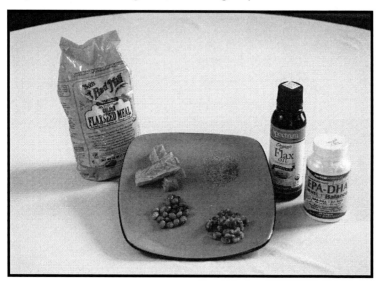

Essential Fats Lower Bad Cholesterol and Increase the Good

Essential fats lower the LDL, "bad" cholesterol in our blood and increase the HDL, "good" cholesterol. The bad cholesterol will grow very quickly when your diet isn't balanced. When bad cholesterol outnumbers the good cholesterol, the bad fat sticks to the artery walls making the passage for blood very narrow. This pressure on the artery walls contributes to an increase in blood pressure. High blood pressure and high cholesterol are both major risk factors for heart disease.

The good cholesterol (HDL) is the enemy of the bad cholesterol (LDL). When you have a lot of these good guys circulating in your blood, they actually remove the bad cholesterol from your body. If you allow your arteries to get clogged with bad cholesterol, your heart is going to get very mad at you, and may decide to stop working. It's not that it wants to. It's just difficult to pump blood through a pin hole.

The good news is that you can reverse this clogged mess when you increase the number of good cholesterol. If you follow the six -step plan, there is a really good chance you will increase the good cholesterol. Three out of the six steps are the ingredients for good cholesterol: fiber, exercise, and essential fats.

Essential Fats Build Brains

Part of the grey matter in your brain is made from essential fats. It started when you were in the womb. Essential fats are significant in growing fetus brain cells. Put in simple language, essential fats build brain cells for growing fetuses, and continue to supply our brain with these needed fats all through our adult life.

For the first time ever in human history, government officials claim our children today will **not** outlive their parents! Not because of war or famine, but because of a lack of balance. It shouldn't be a big surprise that most of the young people on our planet do not eat the correct balance of most foods, and essential fats are at the top of the list. The same studies report essential fat deficiency has been linked to anger, depression and learning behavior in children.

Dr. Daniel G. Amen in his book, *Making a Good Brain Great*, has an entire chapter dedicated to brain food. The lifestyle he advocates is: adequate water, proper portions of protein, and carbohydrates with lots of fiber, essential fats and exercise. Dr. Amen claims these are all the ingredients that make a good brain great, and are the same ones advocated in my six-step plan.

Dr. Amen explains scientifically why and how everything works in the brain the way it does. He states in his book, *"Diet and fish oil help to balance brain function. The nice thing about this approach is that there are no side effects; unlike the medications used to help balance brain functions, which sometimes are clearly needed, diet and fish oil have no downside!"*

Hormone Function

Another major influence these fatty acids have is that they create a group of hormone-like substances called *prostaglandins*. As if brain development, cellular and heart protection weren't enough! Hormones are responsible for controlling just about every bodily function. I think of hormones as the worker-bees. Instead of the raw materials that sit around waiting to be put to good use, these guys actually get the job done! The prostaglandins may be the largest workforce we have on the job, working hard for you!

These hormones have something to do with just about every bodily function. For starters, they regulate blood pressure, nerve transmission, digestive tract, reproductive system, immune systems, allergic and inflammation responses, production of other hormones, and they control fluid pressure in the eyes, ears and joints. What quality of life do you think you'd have if any one of these areas were not working right? How much money do you think you would have to spend to straighten things out? Essential fats keep these hormones working for you so you can have good health and not have to spend a zillion dollars trying to fix problems! The next big question should be, where do they come from and how do you keep them balanced?

Where do These Essential Fats Come From?

Essential fats come from our food. A lack of these vital fats will send you to the hospital, but not right away. It is a slow, agonizing process. You get plenty of warning. The symptoms are usually full blown and in your face. The problem is you're clueless as to what they mean or what to do about it.

The Source of Omga-6 and Omega-3 the Two Major Essential Fats

The essential fats we are referring to are the Omega-6 and Omega-3 fats. In order for these fats to work like they are suppose to, you must eat the proper amounts in the proper balance. If you fail to understand the Omega 3 and Omega 6 connection, then you're more likely to suffer from an imbalance that will create a symptom you may never associate with having a lack of essential fat.

Hopefully by now it should start to be clear that the whole body operates on a system of balance, and essential fats are no different.

Omega-6 fatty acids are the most available. It would be highly unlikely to have a deficiency in these fats. They are in most foods, including animal proteins, vegetables, fruits, nuts, seeds, grains, oils made from grains such as safflower, and corn oils.

Omega-3 fats are much harder to find. They are in cold

water fish, (salmon, halibut, tuna, sardines) flaxseed, and flax oil, and to a lesser extent, pumpkin seeds, walnuts, canola, and olive oil.

What Is The Real Source Of The Omega Fats?

The essential fats Omega-3 and Omega-6 fatty acids, all start out as plants. They have fancy names like Alph-linoleic (Omega-3) and the Linoleic (Omega-6). Animals that eat plant sources of alpha-linoleic and linoleic fats, naturally convert them into Omega-3 and Omega-6 fats. Take for example cold water fish like salmon. They eat rich sources of Alpha-linoleic fats found in spirulina and plankton, which are cold water sea plants. This explains the rich source of Omega-3 fats that we find in fish oil. Not all fish are a rich source of Omega-3 fat, only those that come from cold water and eat plankton and spirulina.

The plants and animals that have Alpha-linoleic (Omega-3 fats) are found in cold climates. If you eat a salmon that has been farmed raised in Chili, you are eating a good source of protein but not Omega-3 fat. Fish from South America are not eating Alpha-linoleic plants only found in cold deep waters like what Alaskan salmon eat.

Omega-6 fats (Liniolec fats) grow in warmer climates, which include just about everything else that comes from a plant, like vegetables, beans, grains, and those animals that eat these foods.

**TWO FACTORS TO BALANCE
OMEGA-3 FATS:**

1. Add Omega-3 Fats to Your Diet
2. Do Not Eat Trans-Fats or
   Hydrogenated Fats

---

1. Add Omega-3 Fats to Your Diet

If the Omega Balance is Wrong, You May be Gone

These essential fats Omega-6 and Omega-3 work in partnership with each other. They need each other in the right amounts and the right ratio to work optimally. If the amount of Omega-6 fat is not at a certain ratio to the Omega-3 fats, then the essential fats are ineffective. It is hard to imagine that you could be deficient in these essential fats when you are eating healthy Omega-6 foods such as: vegetables, chicken, meat, beans, grains, eggs and dairy. The problem is that it has to be a certain ratio (balance) of Omega-3 fats to Omega-6 fats. There is a really good chance you will consume an adequate amount of Omega-6 fats, but not the Omega-3 fats, because they only come from a few sources, such as: cold water fish, certain oils, and select seeds and nuts, so if you do not eat foods with these Omega-3 fats, the ratio is off, and you become deficient in essential fats.

When the Omega-6 fats are in greater number than the Omega-3 fats, the body is unable to absorb Omega-3 fats, the amount of essential fats you end up with is a **big ZERO**. Omega-6 fats by themselves create an imbalance, which causes inflammation, destroying any benefit good fats have on helping you stay healthy. Let me make this very clear. It is worth repeating.

You are deficient in essential fats unless you keep a healthy balance of each, and the only way to do this is to eat foods rich in Omega-3 fat.

The correct ratio is 5 units of Omega-6 fats to 1 unit of Omega-3 fat. This makes it a 5:1 ratio. Let's suppose you are diligent about eating healthy, you consume food from the four basic food groups, grains, vegetables and fruits, beans, dairy and meat, and you limit your processed foods. Although you are eating healthy, your essential fat ratio is 20:1 not the recommended 5:1. Worse yet is if you are like the typical overweight American, and you eat chips, packaged foods that have trans fats, excess animal proteins, and you love your fried food. The ratio in this case is more like 40:1. When you include trans-fats with an already low ratio of Omega-3 fats, you get inflammation that develops symptoms for illness more severe and sooner than the healthier eater. Regardless of whether you are a little sick or a whole lot sick, you are still out of balance, which means your body cannot regulate itself. It really doesn't matter if you have a 20:1 or a 40:1 ratio. Both miss the mark, creating a fatty acid imbalance.

Cardiologists prescribe Omega-3 fats to their patients, because overwhelming research supports that a diet high in Omega-6 fats and low in Omega-3 fats causes inflammation, especially in relation to heart disease. By prescribing

Omega-3 fats, they are trying to balance the ratio, raising the level of Omega-3 fats to offset the high Omega-6 fats that are so prevalent in our food environment.

Heart disease is the number one killer, and the studies show that balancing these fats can actually help **reverse heart disease**. The inflammatory complications from a diet high in animal fats and trans-fats can also affect those who suffer from joint pain. Omega-3 supplementation has become widely accepted as a method of relief for arthritis and other joint aliments.

How to Balance the Essential Fat Ratio
From all the evidence research provides, an essential fat balance is impossible without Omega-3 intervention. With the assault on fats in the American diet, it would be virtually impossible to maintain an adequate ratio of Omega-6 to Omega-3, therefore you have to find ways to include Omega-3 fats in your diet.

Most physicians believe the most optimum dose is 500mg to 2 grams of Omega-3 fats per day for the entire population, with medical supervision for special conditions. Some medical experts claim a more conservative amount of just 2 servings of cold water fish per week will meet the required amount for the average person, which works out to be approximately 2-3 grams per week. But these same experts change their recommendation to 1-2 grams per day if heart disease is present.

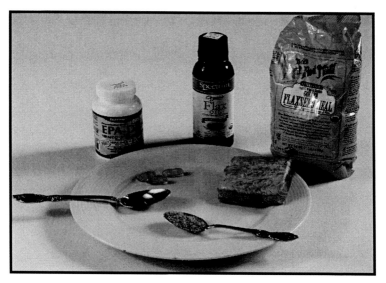

One gram of Omega-3 per day will provide the adequate ratio of fatty acid balance.

One gram per day of Omega-3 fats would equal the following:

1 tsp of ground flax seeds
½ tsp flax oil
2 ounces of wild salmon
1-3 capsules DHA & EPA supplement (varies by brand)

Too Much of a Good Thing Can Be Bad

If you are taking medications or have certain health conditions, you need to be careful when taking an essential fat supplement. Make sure you're under the supervision of a healthcare provider. Type 2 diabetes individuals can have an increase in blood sugar levels, and a diet high in omega-3 fat has shown to decrease blood pressure and thin the blood. Even the amount of cold water fish you eat needs to be monitored by a doctor for people on antico-agulants and blood pressure medication. Omega-3 fatty acids should be used cautiously if you have a bleeding disorder and are taking medication for this. You could be at an increased risk for hemorrhaging.

What Do the Experts Recommend?

According to the National Institute of Health (NIH), at least 2 percent of total daily calories should come from Omega-3 fats. They claim this is the most optimal for the entire population, because of the high risk of imbalance. To meet this recommendation, a person consuming 2,000 calories per day should eat at least 2-3 grams of omega-3 fats from foods.

The Institute of Medicine at the National Academy of Sciences claims the adequate intake for Omega-3 fats is 1.1 grams for female teenagers and 1.6 grams for male teenagers.

The American Heart Association recommends that if you have no history of heart disease, then cold water fish, at least twice a week, is adequate. If you have heart disease, then 1 gram of EPA and DHA is suggested. If you have high blood pressure then 2-4 grams of Omega-3 is best.

All agree for anyone with special needs, especially those with bleeding conditions, should consult a physician.

Digestion and Absorption of Omega-3 Fats

Warning! Some conditions such as diabetes, schizophrenia, and aging can impede the absorption of essential fats. Sometimes certain medical conditions make it difficult for the body to break down essential fats in the plant form. For this special population, the omega source, fish oil, is better absorbed than the plant source of flax seeds or walnuts.

If you don't have any special condition, and you seem to digest nuts and seeds without any problems, there is the added benefit of natural cancer preventive chemicals from the plant source (flax seeds) that you won't find in the fish. There is also a rich source of soluble and insoluble fibers that you won't find in the animal source. So eating the plant source not only provides you with your essential fats, but you get a little extra nutrient boost in the process.

The US Environmental Protection Agency warns us to limit the intake of fish and fish oils because of the possibility of potentially harmful contaminants, such as mercury, that has been detected in sport-caught and commercial fishing. Pregnant and nursing women, young children, and older adults need to avoid eating fish that were found to have higher levels of these toxins, such as swordfish, shark, and mackerel, and to a lesser extent, tuna. Caution should also be taken with fish oil that is unrefined due to pesticides that were found in several of the batches tested.

Omega-3 Supplements

Although you get added nutritional benefits from eating essential fats from their natural food sources, there are those who are unable to eat the seeds and can't take fish oil. For these people supplements become an alternative.

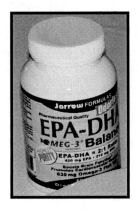

The supplements for essential fats usually come in a gel pill where the essential fats have been broken down into their most simple chemical structure. Having a pill which is already in the form simplest for a cell to accept it means that the body will not have to separate the fiber, carbs, and proteins from the seed. The cell accepts (EPA & DHA), much easier because all the work of breaking it down has been done in a lab. Not that I'm trying to give you a chemistry lesson, but it helps when you go to your local health store to know that a supplement that has EPA & DHA is an essential fatty acid supplement. The EPA and DHA is the simplest form which makes it more advantageous for those with compromised systems due to age or medical conditions because it is easier for the body to absorb the nutrients.

2. Do Not Eat Trans-Fats or Hydrogenated Fats

The whole story on fat can be overwhelming, but I'm going to make it easy. The only fat you need to be very concerned about staying away from are those that are rancid. You would hope people would have enough sense not to eat rancid fat. It doesn't take a heart surgeon to tell you anything rancid in your body will eventually kill you. Well, unfortunately, it is common place in America.

There is a food processing called _hydrogenation_ that makes perfectly good fats rancid. Once rancid, they are referred to as _trans-fats_. It is a laboratory type of controlled rancidity, tasteless, odor-less. You don't even know it's rancid. And, actually, these fats taste great and can be addicting.

Hydrogenated fats are popular with the food industry, as they are helpful in preserving food. Want to know why?

Well, hydrogenation makes the fat bad, so it can't go rancid. In other words, if a fat is already rancid, then it has less opportunity to become rancid on the grocery shelf. Sounds very weird, I know. It took me a while to get it too, but it's part of processed food. Anything in a wrapper needs to stay stable and last a long time on a shelf. Bad fats take a long time to go rancid. Some packaged foods (sugary foods such as cookies, chips, filling cakes, mixes, cereals, pastries), can actually keep stable on a shelf for more than a year. I believe it may have to do with money, because it certainly isn't about our health. Some advocacy groups protested and thought that consumers should know what's in our food. They put a lot of pressure on the government, and in 2006, the food industry was required to list trans fats on the label for all packaged food. Luckily for the food industry, most Americans are fat, tired, and clueless. So, business continues as usual.

Another way to make a good fat rancid is to cook it on high temperatures, like frying or sautéing until it sizzles, and the fat bubbles jump in the pan. Smells great, tastes great, but cooking on high heat turns a good fat into a trans-fat that clogs your arteries and causes inflammation that leads to serious illness like heart disease.

> *The solution for lowering cholesterol or losing weight isn't about eating a certain food or eliminating another. It is about the entire system of balance. These six-steps help get you there. It is not one step but all six steps working together.*

Trans-fat Summary

Trans-fats, hydrogenated monsters, do a real mess-up job on the arteries and raise the fat level in the blood. They make the cells stiff and vulnerable—the opposite of what an essential fat does. Trans-fats destroy the Omega-3 fatty acid balance. Trans-fats destroy the fatty acids needed to break down stored body fat, which makes weight loss difficult. Fried foods or cooking on high heat and the process of hydrogenation create trans-fats. Plain and simple: don't eat them.

Why is Everyone so Worried About Cholesterol?

There is enough conclusive evidence that high cholesterol puts you at risk for heart disease. Anything under 200 milligrams/deciliter and you have nothing to worry about. Go over 240 and you will be on medication.

Low cholesterol isn't good either. Anything under 160 milligrams/deciliter has been linked to Parkinson's, liver cancer, lung and respiratory disease, alcoholism, and depression. Low cholesterol has been associated with aggressive behavior with suicidal tendencies, and it is believed that low levels of cholesterol affect the serotonin levels in the brain, which is a mood enhancer.

Cholesterol is important to our survival. Our body produces it for a reason. It does a lot of good like regulating the body's use of calcium, fat digestion, nerve function, and creating sex hormones and cortisone.

Once again, cholesterol is about maintaining a balance of good cholesterols (HDL) to bad cholesterols (LDL). To eat saturated fats found in dairy, eggs, and butter should not be a problem if you maintain balance with essential fats, fiber, carb, proteins and exercise. Eating healthy has less to do with lowering cholesterol and everything to do with balance. If you keep everything else balanced, cholesterol is rarely a problem.

Include 1-2 grams of Omega-3 fats in your daily diet, know what foods have them.

Food	One gram omega-3
Flax seeds (ground)	1 tsp
Flax oil	½ tsp
Cod liver oil	1 Tablespoon
Fish oil	1 Tablespoon
Canola Oil (cold pressed)	4 Tablespoons
Olive Oil (extra virgin)	4 Tablespoons
Wild salmon	2 ounces
Scallops	½ cup
Halibut	8 ounces
Tuna	8 ounces
Walnuts	4 whole (¼ cup pieces)
Pumkin Seeds	1/3 cup
Tofu	8 ounces
Soybeans	1 cup
Beans (most varities)	3 cups

Moving Forward

Up to this point we have focused mostly on information regarding balance, educating you on how to keep your body properly regulated, so you are able to rewire your brain. Now we need to start looking at how to apply this balance into your life. The next few chapters are more about applying balance to your life. Portion sizes are where we kick start the application process of balance.

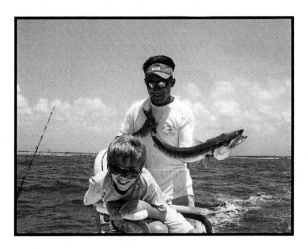

Gavin Haag not sure if this catch is a keeper

NINE

PORTION SIZES

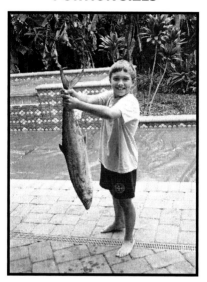

Hopefully Gavin's portion size is less than his catch

Don't Cut Portions

How many times have you heard that to lose weight, all you need to do is cut portion sizes in half? That being overweight is the result of eating too much, and if you can somehow shrink your stomach and train yourself to eat less, then you will no longer have a problem? This is a weight-loss myth and a ridiculous statement! I'm going to prove to you that cutting portion sizes in half could lead to obesity and malnutrition, and it could be one of the dumbest approaches to weight loss ever!

Before you can really understand why this is a crazy theory (and why it ticks me off, big time), you need to take a look at what a portion size means to you personally, your body, the food industry, your local restaurant, and the so-called experts in the field of healthy eating and weight loss.

What a Portion Size Means to You

Your doctor tells you to cut down on your portion sizes to lose weight. Sounds great, but how can you lower your portion sizes when you're starving? That is the way it will feel after two-to-three days of restricting your calories. Eating large portions seems justified when you have hardly eaten all day.

No one likes to feel hungry. It is the number one (and probably number two, three, and four) reason why people don't stay on diets. Hunger is your body's way of telling you that you need food. The signal for more food can happen for many reasons. Many times it is not because we are truly hungry, at least in the sense that we need food for nutrition and fuel.

Many times we eat because we are bored, or we feel it is time to eat, for entertainment purposes. Or we eat because we are suffering from a sugar addiction and our hormones trigger us to eat more. We also use food as a drug to relieve stress. Large portions create a calming effect that seems to be a perfect solution to a long, stressful day. Eating large portions also serves as a sedative, a calming drug. It is a way of checking out of your current situation and providing an escape for a brief period. You become lethargic, barely moving physically or mentally, because you are emotionally numb. After time, you can begin to look forward to that calm, relaxed feeling that masks emotions that are anything but. You may not realize that what you are feeling is not hunger. It is more like an urge or need to eat. And it's more than just providing nutrition. For some, it becomes a lover, an entertainment, a drug.

When this mindless comfort eating is the one thing in life that really brings you joy, you and everyone who looks at you knows there is a problem. Sure, you have become dependant on the checking-out, calming effect. The problem is that along with that relaxed calming effect, you feel bloated, embarrassed about how fat you have become, and you feel tired most of the next day. You wish you could stop, but you feel trapped.

You Can Break Free

Eating large portions of comforting food always feels good during the act of consuming, but it never feels good to live with yourself after. Being fat makes you feel bad, not just physically but emotionally. You depend on those huge portions, and they can manifest themselves into a real physical need. What starts out as a coping strategy can turn into a full blown food addiction, and you begin to spin out of control, fixing your problem with the very thing that is causing it.

Before you can break yourself of this cycle, you have to have an understanding of what is going on inside your brain and your body, as well as what is going on around you, and your food environment.

The Body Knows Only Immediate Needs

Your body is constantly working 24 hours, seven days a week. There is no "on" or "off" switch. Cells are dying and rebuilding every second of the day. As long as you are breathing, the body never rests, and is in constant motion. This is why our bodies need raw materials, in small amounts, all day long. It doesn't fix the immune system at 3:00 in the afternoon or only absorb protein at 6:00 in the morning so it can repair muscle tissue. The body is fixing the immune system and repairing muscle tissue every minute of the day!

Luckily, your body keeps reserves of resources to pull from. The problem is that for many nutrients, the reserve may only last anywhere from 3-24 hours. Ideally, your body would like for you to consume nutrients at the same rate you expend them, never allowing your reserves to dwindle down or become empty. But this is not a realistic scenario. What typically happens is that your body gets what it can from the foods you eat and then compromises in areas it has to. You have no awareness that the body needs raw materials, and to go without, means stealing from your own body tissue. Or even worse, your body not being able to do its job at all, which results in poor health. **Instead, you get a surplus of calories while your cells starve for needed nutrients.**

You have no way of communicating to your body when the next meal is coming, or what you will be having. Let's take protein, for example. If the body needs to fix muscle tissue at 3:00 in the afternoon, and the protein reserves are empty, the body has no way of knowing that at 6:00 p.m., you plan to feast on a 10-ounce tenderloin. The body works on demand, using what it needs, at the time it needs it. And, yes, that includes stealing protein from your own muscle tissue. At 3:00 in the afternoon, your upper arm or thigh muscle becomes the tenderloin meal for a hungry body in need of raw materials.

How Your Body Sees a Portion Size

The body determines a good portion size based on what it needs at that particular moment. If you just exercised hard for one hour, your body will use a different portion size than if you just woke from a nap.

It is in need of raw materials to build and repair cells and optimum fuel for energy. When your body is hungry (not to be confused with food addiction from an imbalance, but true hunger), it is telling you that this is the best time to get some really important work done. Your body is saying, *"Give me the raw materials I need now, so I can give you an awesome body later."* Ignore the body's request, and it will improvise, putting you in survival mode. You can expect your metabolism to slow down, for your cells to steal nutrients from other, healthier cells, and the entire health of your body to become compromised.

Now that you understand that, think how dumb it is to take an appetite suppressant for weight loss, so you won't be reminded that the body is trying to keep you alive!

Why Appetite Suppressants Don't Work

Appetite suppressants kill any communication your body has with your brain to get what it needs to stay healthy and energetic. Appetite suppressants are usually accompanied by stimulants. This way, you can wipe out your adrenal glands while starving your cells, lose weight, and have access to this hyper-nervous energy, all in one sweep. Five years later, when you are sick as a dog, obese, and unable to lose a pound, and no one knows why, you can reflect back on your skinny hyper days, when you were a skinny waif living off appetite suppressants and stimulants.

Ideally, a good portion should be your response to the body's request for food; at least this is how your body sees it. It has an investment in your survival, and it would like for you to be smart, starting with raw materials that it can use to repair, build, and fuel itself.

From your body's perspective, hunger is its way of telling you it needs nutrients, not just food to fill your gut or some worthless morsel that serves no other purpose but to pacify the request. Think of it this way: the body has to shift through all the calories to find anything of value. When you eat empty calories, it is a major disappointment. This is kind of like getting a beautifully wrapped present with nothing inside.

Cutting Portions Can Cut Nutrients

Suppose you eat the typical American diet that provides double the calories but half of the needed nutrients. Now imagine cutting that in half! Your calories may be in line, but the nutrients are not. When most people think of cutting portion sizes, they think of cutting back on calories. Experts tell us that if we eat fewer calories, we lose weight, which is half true. It is true that if you eat less than you consume, you lose weight, but if you are not balanced or nutritional in the process, you won't last long. Eventually, you will gain weight, because your body will demand more food, which will result in you consuming twice your daily requirement of calories. The real tragedy is that you may not even get a portion that is worth a darn in the process.

Your body hopes you will not let calories or the bulk of food be the determining factor for portion size. From your body's perspective, portion size has very little to do with the amount of food on a plate or the number of calories on a label, but rather how many nutrients are in those calories, and what it can actually do with those nutrients. **Studies show that if you give your body all the nutrients it needs by maintaining protein, fiber, carbohydrate, and essential fat requirements, while keeping hormonal balance in the process, then your body will naturally cut your portion sizes for you.** You will feel satisfied on less food. Your body won't be screaming for more calories. Portion sizes are important but it only works when you can analyze what makes a good portion size and apply those rules to your life. If not, you will overeat, get fat, and may not even be healthy in the process.

How the Food Industry Sees a Portion Size

The food industry determines a serving size by giving us a caloric value. All labels have the calories for one serving as well, as the total number of servings in the package. This calorie value is a random number the food manufacturer decided a single serving should be. According to the food industry, one serving size is an average of 150-250 calories. Recently, though, 100-calorie serving snacks have entered the market. As if eating less of a certain food will fix the problem. All it really does is make us want three or four servings of the 100-calorie snack.

Studies show people who trust their bodies to food establishments and the food industry tend to be obese, depressed, and have a lack of energy. Keep in mind that eating establishments and the food industry do not view a portion size with the same interest as your body does. If they did, we wouldn't have an obesity epidemic in this country.

Does the food industry honestly believe that eating smaller portions of 100-calorie nutritionally inadequate snacks is the answer? They still want you to believe that a portion size is only about calories, and the reason why Americans are fat is that they lack self control and are unable to monitor portion sizes. Not so.

The Potato Chip Dilemma

Take, for example, one serving size of potato chips at 180 calories for one serving, which is only 10-12 chips. If you eat 20-24 chips, you have had 2 portions of food, according to the food industry label, but your body sees only empty calories. There are no real portions of any value in the food industry's two servings of potato chips. If you are hungry enough, you could easily eat three or four servings of potato chips at a whopping 400-500 calories and have still provided no nutritional portions to your body.

At 500 calories, the food industry label claims that you have had three servings of food. Your body tells you that you have had none. It is still hungry, still searching for quality portions of food, and you consume double the calories. What this means is that you can eat 500 calories and 20 minutes later, still feel hungry. If you had given your body 500 calories of nutrient-rich food, you would feel satisfied and might not need to eat for several hours.

How the US Government Sees a Portion Size

On the other hand, the government, a highly respected panel of experts, knows exactly what a serving size should be for good health. It describes a healthy diet through dietary guidelines categorized in food groups. It uses a colorful pyramid chart recommending the amount of food you need from each group. The food groups emphasize fruits, vegetables, whole grains, milk products, meat, beans, and oils. You can go on their website **www.mypyramid.gov** and learn about the food groups.

They mention calories, of course, in regard to weight management, explaining to the public that if input of calories exceeds output, weight gain is expected. What these experts are very clear about is that they don't use calories to measure a portion size because they know this is ridiculous and has no relevancy to good health or weight loss. The U. S. My Pyramid program bases portion sizes on food groups, not calories.

How a Restaurant Sees a Portion Size

Restaurants sell entertainment, taste, and cost value through the commodity of food. This is the criteria used for most restaurants in determining portion sizes. Restaurants are in the business of making money, your body is in the business of health, and for most of us, our brains are clueless! We let our hormones and emotions think for us. Many restaurants sell food based on cost value. They give you a lot of calories for your buck. We wouldn't buy these calories unless they tasted great, in a pleasant, entertaining environment. How hard do you think it is to make cheap food taste great? I'll give you a hint…very easy. Add sugar, salt, and fat, and it will be pretty darn irresistible. Thanks to technology and processing, there is an abundance of low-quality food, sold in bulk, priced fairly cheap.

There are enough calories in one menu entree to supply enough calories for the entire day, with less than one quarter of your daily nutritional requirement. From your body's viewpoint, this is a hostile environment, and the only hope is that you will have the brains to figure it out.

Smart Portions Versus Small Portions

Everyone agrees on one truth: If portion sizes are smaller, resulting in our eating less, then weight loss is inevitable. If this becomes a lifestyle, then weight gain is not part of that lifestyle. The problem is that if portions are solely based on cutting back calories, or if you feel deprived as if you are being forced to cut back, this doesn't work. Your body will fight back, and in the end, you will be the loser.

Less calories through smaller portions has to be something your body is in total agreement with, and it has to be a natural process. The problem is that our current food environment doesn't allow this natural process to occur because they are not offering us smart food. This means you are going to have to use your brain to help your body. Remember, your body will not be able to do this on its own. It reacts to what you feed it and then, you become a victim of its reaction.

Naturally Satisfied

If your body has everything it needs and there are no food addiction triggers, then it will naturally feel satisfied. If you can figure out how to eat a smart portion, your body will regulate your desire for more food; you will get more energy and be much healthier for it. Eating smart portions allows your body to automatically regulate portion sizes for you. A smart portion is when the body receives nutrients, without any addiction triggers, and with no excess calories

TWO FACTS ABOUT SMART PORTIONS

1. Smart portions contain no extra empty calories.

2. Smart portions meet the body's need for raw materials while maintaining balance.

1. Smart Portions Contain No Extra Empty Calories

Excess calories are what make us fat. If every time you ate, there were only enough calories to take care of business, then you would never have to worry about gaining weight. Most people laugh at the thought that this could be possible, convinced it isn't realistic. Actually, your body would prefer a smart portion with no excess calories that need to be stored as fat. Remember, obesity is a burden on your body. **A life-threatening one.**

Your body isn't really looking for extra calories. The extra calories just happen to be the end result. Your body is searching for raw materials and because you don't know what a smart portion is, you eat a lot of excess calories in the process. Think of a single serving of food from a food manufacturer. Your body is looking for nutrients, not calories. As for a restaurant, you don't know if they have added 300-400 extra calories of butter to one serving of fish you think is only 200 calories.

Hormones

Even if you ate the exact calories with all the needed nutrients, and there was nothing left over to be stored as body fat, you could still have huge swings in your hormones. You can still have an imbalance in your carbohydrate reserve and trigger a hormonal response eating healthy nutrient rich foods.

It is ridiculous to think you can just cut your portions in half. The body will demand more food that will most likely not be balanced resulting in hormonal swings. This is less about hunger and more about addiction. Keeping calories low has everything to do with being smart. Remember, the body works on an *as-needed basis* and eating smart is realizing the body's **current** needs. Every time you eat, your body takes what it needs at that particular moment and gets rid of the excess. If you eat more nutrients or calories than the body needs, it discards the excess nutrients in your urine and stores any excess calories as fat.

Welcome to Your Blubber

Let's suppose you binge on 1,000 calories, but your body has immediate needs for only 400 calories. This means that 400 calories are delivered to the muscles for fuel and nutrition, leaving more than half of the remaining calories stored as body fat. Any nutrients your body didn't use at the time of consumption are discarded. That's right. Raw materials the body doesn't need are eliminated and the extra fuel is stored as body fat. Most people do not realize that fat is just stored blubber that has no nutritional value because anything that was worth a darn was either used or discarded at the time of consumption.

Body fat's sole purpose is to provide enough fuel to keep you alive. The excess body fat that is sitting on hips legs, and stomach has no nutritional value. If you ever have to live off your fat, as in the case of a restricted weight-loss program, you will be malnourished, and feel miserable. Expect your hair to fall out, skin problems, fatigue and ill health, all from lack of nutrients. These programs may appear to solve short-term weight-loss problems, but in the long run, you will be the real loser. Bottom line, eventually it will come down to learning the lifestyle that will keep you lean and healthy.

Eating smaller amounts of food keeps calories lower and it would appear to be the answer. This may make good sense but, unfortunately, it will not work by itself. The body needs raw materials to function. Just eating small amounts with no regard to what the body needs to keep you alive doesn't solve anything. In fact, you will feel hungry all of the time and never be satisfied. Trying to eat smaller portions for weight maintenance will be torture. Smart portions need to have nutrients to keep your hormones and protein and carbohydrate reserves balanced.

Smart portion sizes should come as close as possible to the number of calories and nutrients the body needs at that immediate moment. If you do it right, this means no excess calories are available to be stored as fat and everything gets put to good use. It should make sense that portion sizes depend on what you are doing that particular day. The more active you are, the larger the portion sizes you can afford without fat storage. My six-step plan is about learning to create smart portions with foods you select. After all, it is your lifestyle.

2. Smart Portions Meet the Body's Need for Raw Materials While Maintaining Balance

Your body is doing millions of small jobs simultaneously all day long. Therefore, it would make sense that it needs small amounts of nutrients as it is working. From the body's perspective, the sole purpose of eating is to provide needed materials to keep you moving, thinking and breathing.

The reality is that most of us have no idea what foods do for us. We eat carelessly when we are hungry and trust food establishments and the food industry to look out for us, and then are shocked when we are fat, tired, and sick.

Smart portions need to supply the body with these needed materials to get all the millions of jobs done. Vitamins, minerals, enzymes, protein, fiber, carbohydrates, omega-3 fats, are all part of that requirement.

What Makes a Smart Portion?

1. Smart portions include complete protein reserves that are adequate for your body mass.

The body needs protein to build and repair tissue. Make sure you are getting the right amount of protein, at the right time in the right combinations for your body size. Too much protein or not enough are both bad for your health.

2. Smart portions do not allow carbohydrate reserves to become depleted or cause hormonal havoc.

Manage your carbohydrate reserves by knowing how many carbs you need. Remember, if your carbohydrate reserves are allowed to become depleted, even a small amount of a high sugary carbohydrate will trigger an episode of binging that will result in insulin imbalances and create an addictive cycle. Too much sugar at one time, even when it is from a healthy source, can cause a hormonal roller coaster.

3. Smart portions include good fats, not bad fats.

Portions that have bad fats throw off the essential fatty acid balance, which means *essential fats no longer function as they should. This has a negative effect on inflammation and the hormonal regulatory process. Obesity and disease are affiliated with essential fat imbalances. Smart portions do not include trans-fats, but do include Omega-3 fats.*

Long Periods Between Meals Creates Imbalance.

Five or six hours without food and your body is not balanced. Think of it this way, after a period of deprivation any food is good food. The body wants the quickest and most food possible. When you eat less frequently, such as one or two times a day, you will need a ton of willpower to make smart choices. Just a small serving of 200 calories between meals of protein and fiber can be enough to keep the body from falling into the starvation trap where meals turn into feasts of all the wrong foods.

How Do I Apply These Smart Portions?

Now that you have the information and you're ready to make smart choices, you need a tool to help you apply this information to your life. Tools are not the end-all. They should only serve as instruments to help us reach our goals. Tools by themselves are not effective unless you know how and why to use them. The tool that can help you, and has helped thousands of others just like you, is the **200-calorie tool.** This tool enables you to look at food and know if it is a balanced choice, which in turn, makes it the *smartest choice.*

The Truth About Portions

If you eat less you weigh less. The problem is smaller portions are an impossible lifestyle of torture and deprivation because you are eating less of an already inadequate portion and your body fights back by overeating.

If you pick quality proteins and fibers, and include omega-3 fats into your diet, you have a much better chance of providing your body what it needs. What makes healthy choices become smart choices is your ability to balance these foods.

The Six Step process teaches you how to balance portions where eating less happens naturally because the body is satisfied.

Being balanced is the only way to control portions.

TEN

THE 200-CALORIE RULE

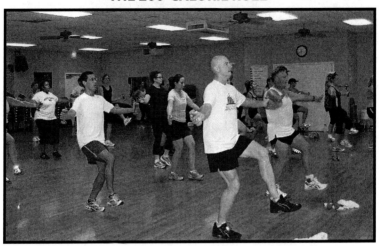

Myrna's aerobic class in Tampa Florida

The 200-calorie rule is used to determine a quick nutritional balance for food using the food label to compare one serving of calories to protein and fiber. The key is to try and keep a **minimum** of **8 grams of protein** and **4 grams of fiber** for every 200-calorie portion.

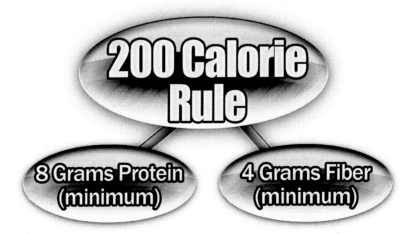

Why 200 Calories?

The 200-calorie tool uses 200 calories as a caloric value in determining the protein-fiber combinations. Here's why. Two hundred calories seems to be the middle of the road for most single servings according to the food industry. The food label's description of a serving size is anywhere from 150-250 calories, so I am just averaging here.

Nutrition Facts

Serving Size 1/2 cup (about 82g)
Servings Per Container 8

Amount Per Serving

Calories 200   Calories from Fat 130

	% Daily Value*
Total Fat 14g	22%
Saturated Fat 9g	45%
Trans Fat 0g	
Cholesterol 55mg	18%
Sodium 40mg	2%
Total Carbohydrate 17g	6%
Dietary Fiber 1g	4%
Sugars 14g	
Protein 3g	

Vitamin A 10%	•	Vitamin C 0%
Calcium 10%	•	Iron 6%

*Percent Daily Values are based on a 2,000 calorie diet. Your daily values may be higher or lower depending on your calorie needs:

	Calories	2,000	2,500
Total Fat	Less than	65g	80g
Saturated Fat	Less than	20g	25g
Cholesterol	Less than	300mg	300 mg
Sodium	Less than	2,400mg	2,400mg
Total Carbohydrate		300g	375g
Dietary Fiber		25g	30g

Calories per gram:
Fat 9 • Carbohydrate 4 • Protein 4

The 200-calorie figure, being a round number, makes calculations easier when trying to figure it out in your head. The grocery store can turn into a nightmare. It's confusing with food claims, low-fat, all natural, optimum health written all over the packaging. This tool helps you decide what foods make the cart and which ones stay on the shelf.

*Note. The 200-calorie rule doesn't mean that every portion needs to be 200 calories. It is just a tool that

helps you figure out the value and balance of foods at a certain caloric value to know if it is a smart choice.

How it Works

Assume a portion size is 200 calories. Keep in mind that one meal can be 3-4 portion sizes at 600-800 calories, and one snack can be less than one portion, such as 170 calories as in the example of an apple and slice of cheese. **By maintaining a minimum of 8 grams of protein and 4 grams of fiber for every 200 calories, you slow absorption of sugars and provide protein for needed maintenance.** Foods that are slightly less in fiber and protein may be healthy, but still can be risky in maintaining overall balance. It is difficult to find foods that meet the balance on their own, such as a piece of fruit or a slice of bread. Thus we need to combine certain foods to get this ratio to work.

Whether you are consuming 800 calories or 150 calories, a smart portion is determined by estimating its balance. The 200-calorie tool helps you determine the balance of food by estimating the amount of protein and fiber in that one serving. If you eat two or three servings, it is really easy to make the adjustments. I will show you how.

The 200 calorie rule makes grocery shopping a lot easier when trying to make a quick smart decision and the only thing you need to know is the serving size and the amount of protein, fiber, carbohydrates and fats.

Combine food to make smart portions.

Example 1	Calories	Protein	Fiber
3 ounces Turkey	150	22	0
1 whole wheat wrap	200	5	8
Lettuce, tomato, mustard	10	0	2
1 fruit	50	0	4
Total value	**400**	**27**	**13**

Based on the 200 calorie rule, example 1 snack at 27 grams protein and 13 grams fiber for 400 calories would keep you balanced. It has more protein and fiber than the minumum 8 grams protein and 4 grams fiber.

Example 2	Calories	Protein	Fiber
Whole wheat wrap	220	5	8
Hummus, ½ cup	130	8	8
Sprouts, olives tomatoes	50	3	2
Total value	**400**	**16**	**18**

Example 2 has the minimum amount of protein and plenty of fiber for 400 calories to be balanced.

Example 3	Calories	Protein	Fiber
1 cup beans	220	16	16
½ cup rice	100	2	0
Total value	**320**	**18**	**16**

At 320 calories with 18 grams of protein and 16 grams of fiber, example 3 is a smart choice because it is higher than the suggested amount of protein and fiber based on the 200 calorie rule.

Example 4	Calories	Protein	Fiber
Apple	80	0	4
1 ounce cheese	90	7	0
Total value	**170**	**7**	**4**

Although example 4 is a smaller portion, it is still balanced.

Example 5	Calories	Protein	Fiber
¾ cup granola	350	8	6
½ cup milk	70	4	0
½ banana	30	0	2
Total value	**450**	**12**	**8**

Although Example 5 has healthy ingredients, it does not supply enough protein and fiber to keep balance.

Example 5 is a Healthy Snack

...but does not provide the minimum amount of protein and fiber to be balanced. There is not enough protein and fiber to balance the carbohydrates. This meal could trigger an insulin reaction or a binge for more carbs. Although this has plenty of calories, there isn't enough value of nutrients in the calories to satisfy your body. Therefore, you will be hungry within an hour and want more calories.

Example #5 and Applying How it Works

You pick up a box of granola, which is healthy. It advertises it has omega-3 fats and it is the low-sugar variety. Granola is surely a healthier food choice than a processed sugary cereal. But food nutrients are just one criteria in determining a smart portion. You also must consider hormonal balance and excess calories. You find this label shows one serving at 175 calories with 4 grams protein and 3 grams fiber. According to the 200-calorie tool, you realize you need a minimum of 8 grams of protein and 4 grams of fiber. You notice that the 1/3 cup serving only has 175 calories with not enough protein and fiber, so you decide to have two portions at 350 calories thinking this will give you more protein and fiber. Two portions now give you 8 grams of protein and 6 grams of fiber, which is more than before, but not enough to balance the high calories. In other words, your body got one portion of nutritive value with two portions worth of calories. If you used the 200 calorie rule, 350 calories would require double the protien and fiber to be balanced.

This is not saying that granola is a bad food. It is just, at these values, you would be getting extra calories that could cause some hormonal swings, because the fiber and protein are not high enough to slow down the absorption of the carbohydrates, even with the milk. Let's suppose you added a ½ scoop of whey protein and ½ cup of high fiber (Fiber One cereal), and cut back on the granola. This would make your meal balanced, and you would be less hungry, and feel more satisfied.

Example 5 Revised	Calories	Protein	Fiber
½ cup granola	250	6	4
½ cup Fiber Cereal	70	2	5
whey protein ½ scoop	40	10	0
½ cup milk	70	4	0
½ banana	30	0	2
Total value	**460**	**22**	**11**

When example 5 is revised to include more protein and fiber in the mix it becomes a smart choice.

Healthy Portions Versus Balanced Portions

What makes a food healthy depends on what it does for you specifically in regards to balance and nutritional value. Even if food is healthy and keeps you balanced you must also concider if the food agrees with you. How you feel after eating certain foods is a good indication of knowing if that food agrees with you or not. Food intolerances, allergies and diabetes are just a few examples of dietary challenges that require additional research and help from a medical professional. The positive effects of keeping your food balance are destroyed if you have adverse reactions to certain foods.

After taking special dietary needs into concideration, the six-step process helps you decide what foods make up smart portions. By following the six- step process, you allow your body to regulate itself, so you can think smart. This is a lifestyle, not a diet. You empower yourself by learning the rules and using the tools. The six-step process slowly changes your lifestyle. You begin to make healthier choices without feeling as if you have to because you are more in control.

Cheeseburger Slip and Fall

Let's suppose you treat yourself to a cheeseburger, fries and soda. At 1,150 calories, you consumed more than half of your day's worth of calories. Based on the 200-calorie tool, for 1,150 calories it would be smart to consume 48 grams of protein and 24 grams of fiber. Based on what you know in regard to smart portions, it is obvious you had a slip and fall. Your cheeseburger choice has less than 20 grams of protein and 2 grams of fiber.

What makes this slip and fall scenario so challenging, is not the lack of nutrients, but the addictive mindless eating trap you fall into. You will find yourself hungry within two to three hours, and your desire for nourishment will be from the same food source that got you into trouble in the first place.

Don't beat yourself up over it. You have the next meal to redeem yourself, but ask yourself why? How close were you to the six-step process? Chances are, food addiction got the best of you.

I can promise, if you consumed 48 grams of protein and 24 grams of fiber for the same 1,150 calories, you would not be hungry for at least four to six hours, and that is assuming you could eat that much quantity of food at one sitting. The extra bonus is that you would be balanced; therefore, your emotions and hormones wouldn't dictate your next meal.

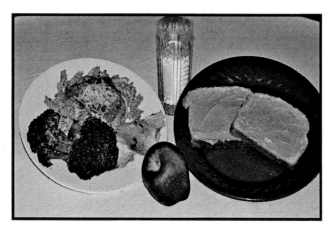

This is what 1,150 calories of smart portions looks like, compared with a cheeseburger, fries, and a cola.

Smart Portion	Calories	Protein	Fiber
1 cup broccoli	50	2	4
1 cup whole wheat pasta	220	14	16
3/4 cup tomato sauce	150	4	3
2 tablespoons cheese	30	2	0
3 ounces chicken	180	20	0
1 apple	80	0	4
1 tablespoon peanut butter	200	4	0
2 slices whole wheat bread	190	4	2
1 cup milk	150	6	0
Total value	**1,150**	**56**	**29**

Compare

Cheese burger fries and cola	Calories	Protein	Fiber
Cheeseburger, special sauce	600	20	0
Lettuce, tomato & onion	10	0	2
Fries	350	0	0
Cola	200	0	0
Total value	**1,150**	**20**	**2**

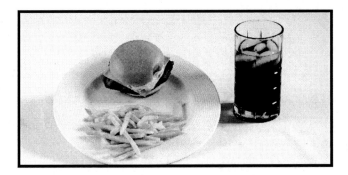

The smart portion has double the volume of food and nutrition versus the cheeseburger.

Think how full you would feel with the smart portion, and how the cheeseburger meal leaves room for dessert.

Low-calorie, low-nutrition snacks serve no purpose

Low- 100-calorie snack

Calories	Protein	Fiber	Fiber
100	2	1	0

Low Calories Do Not Define a Smart Portion.

Do not be fooled into believing this is all there is. It is _not just about calories_, and it is _not just about your weight_. This is a cycle of abuse you are fooled into believing, and it makes you a perfect candidate for media manipulation, food addiction, poor health, fatigue and obesity. Obesity is a hardship on the body, a lifestyle we are forced into because of our lack of awareness on how to be smart.

Brian's set-point theory sets him back

Brian is convinced his body's natural set point at 40 years old is 50 pounds more than what he weighed in his twenties. First of all, studies have disproven the set-point theory. There is no such theory where our body has a set point that makes us predestined to weigh 50 pounds and become obese. There _is_ such a thing as body types, some more curvy than others, but there is no way our body wants us to be fat and toxic. If you think about it, it is stressful and a lot of work for the body to maintain more flesh and clean out more toxins than it has to.

What has Brian so convinced that the set-point theory must be true, is that no matter how much he loses, or how many times he diets, he eventually goes back to his pre-diet weight. He eats organic, mostly vegan food, which convinces him even more that it must be him and can't be the food. By most peoples' standards, he eats obnoxiously healthy, and always gets a clean bill of health from his doctor. Still, his out-of-control eating triggered the food addiction that resulted in his weight gain. Brian is eating healthy, but he isn't eating smart. The 200-calorie tool would help him keep all those whole-grain, organic ingredients of his balanced. This tool will also help his body naturally regulate portions. Eating healthy food all day serves the purpose of supplying the body needed nutrients, but the excess calories, regardless of how healthful they are, will be stored as body fat. This leads to obesity, confirming that healthy portions need to be smart portions.

When Does the 200-calorie Rule Not Apply?

If you are an athlete or lead a physically active lifestyle, you could use anywhere from 800-1,500 calories just to fuel your activity. In this case, pure carbohydrates are your best choice, and the fiber and protein may inhibit the process of carbohydrate absorption during exercise.

When The 200 Calorie Rule Doesn't Apply

When physically active, the muscles need immediate fuel, so the body can deliver sugar to the working muscles. For example, during exercise, the smartest food choices are foods that have carbohydrates that can quickly be delivered to working muscles. The only time insulin will not react to pure sugar is when you are exercising. Insulin doesn't treat sugar the same when eaten during exercise. In fact, the body would rather not have to mess with trying to digest fiber, protein or fats. It prefers to have food quickly leave the digestive tract. In other words, your body wants to focus on working muscles not digesting foods.

Example of Daily Schedule of Carbohydrate Grams

You can see that most of your carbohydrates are centered around activity.

Oatmeal
1/2 cup milk
1 fruit

45 grams carbs

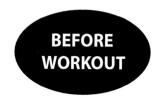

1 Energy bar

45 grams carbs

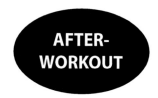

1 cup whole wheat
pasta
2 oz chicken
1/2 cup tomato sauce
60 grams carbs

The rest of the day… the 200 Calorie Rule applies

Exercise Exception

The 200-calorie rule works great in maintaining your regular daily schedule, but during exercise, you want to consume carbohydrates that can immediately supply the muscle with fuel. Therefore, it is best not to have too much protein or fiber during exercise.

Compare Smart Portions to Dumb Portions

Smart Portions	Dumb Portions
Less calories	Double the calories than smart portions
More volume of food	Less volume of food
More nutrition	Empty calories
High fiber	Little fiber
Follows the 200 calorie tool	Doesn't follow the 200 calorie tool
Feel satisfied not full	Feel full not satisfied

Angel Eats Protein and Fiber with no Calorie Limit

Angel can't understand why she's overweight. She insists that she follows the six-step program. Although she has lost 40 pounds, made significant improvements in her diet, and has more energy than a woman half her age, she still can't seem to lose the last 30 pounds. Angel hasn't made the effort of consciously evaluating the caloric value of the protein-fiber combinations she consumes. She hasn't really analyzed her portions. Once she is willing to accept what a smart portion really is and uses the 200 calorie rule, the 30 pounds will melt off.

Smart Portion

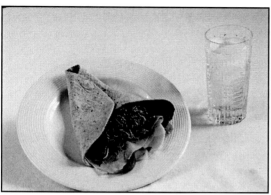

Ham Wrap	Calories	Protein	Fiber
High fiber/lo-cal wrap	100	7	9
2 ounces ham	150	14	0
1 ounce cheese	100	7	0
½ tomato	10	1	1
½ cup sprouts	10	2	3
Total	**370**	**30**	**13**

Dumb Portion

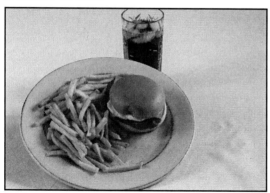

Chicken Sandwich	Calories	Protein	Fiber
Fried Chicken Cheese Special Sauce	600	20	0
1 cup French fries	400	2	1
Soft drink	150	0	0
Total	**1,150**	**22**	**1**

Smart Portion

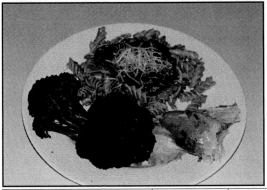

Chicken & Pasta	Calories	Protein	Fiber
1 cup whole wheat pasta	200	7	7
¼ cup tomato sauce and cheese	100	2	1
3 ounces chicken	180	21	0
2 cups brocoli	20	2	8
Total	**500**	**30**	**16**

Dumb Portion

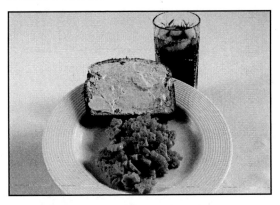

Mac and Cheese	Calories	Protein	Fiber
1 ½ Cup Macaroni and Cheese	400	7	0
Bread	80	2	2
Butter	100	0	0
Soft Drink	150	0	0
Total	**730**	**9**	**2**

Smart Portion

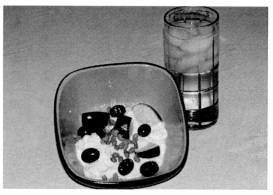

Fruit Bowl	Calories	Protein	Fiber
½ Cup Cottage Cheese	100	15	0
1 cup fruit	50	0	4
2 Tablespoons soy nuts	50	4	3
Total	**200**	**19**	**7**

Dumb Portion

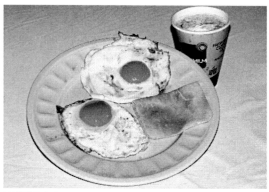

Ham and Eggs	Calories	Protein	Fiber
2 fried eggs	180	14	0
2 ounces ham	150	14	0
Coffee drink	250	7	0
Total	**580**	**35**	**0**

Smart Portion

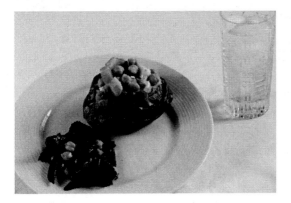

Baked Potato Snack	Calories	Protein	Fiber
Potato	150	2	2
½ cup garbanzo beans	100	7	6
⅓ cup cottage cheese	100	7	0
½ tomato	10	1	1
½ cup sprouts	10	2	3
Total	**370**	**30**	**13**

Dumb Portion

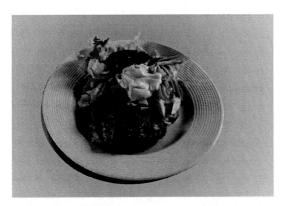

Salad and Chicken	Calories	Protein	Fiber
1 large chicken breast	350	35	0
Salad and tomato, 2 T dressing	150	14	0
Total	**570**	**36**	**3**

Smart Day

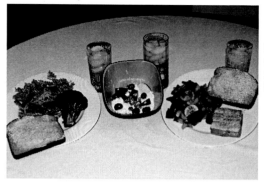

High protein, high fiber, meets carb and protein reserve, balances omega 3 fats.

Diet Dumb Day

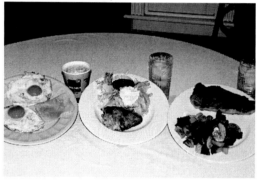

High protein, low fiber depletes carb reserve; has more omega-6 fats than omega-3 fats; promotes acidity and inflamation.

Really Dumb Day

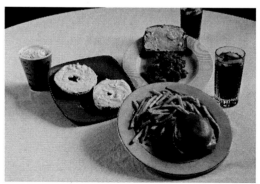

Low protein, low fiber, trans-fats; carb reserves are adequate but process carbs create an addiction where the only foods you want to eat are those that are the least healthy.

Eat Smart... Be Smart

This is a process, not a diet, which means at this point, you are acquiring knowledge and building valuable resources that you will be able to apply. The key is that you know how to choose smart portion sizes based on what to eat, when, and why. If you understand the concept behind a smart portion, you will be able to apply it to your life.

Your body is a machine that you are responsible for maintaining. You cannot be expected to manage a machine that you have little information about. Remember, you live in an environment that thrives on your failure versus your success. The diet industry, food industry, and medical industry depend on your failure.

The government actually wants you to succeed because they are broke and tired of paying the bill for those who are unable, but Washington is filled with lobbyists from the food industry, diet industry, and medical industry who have billions of dollars and can buy influence. So the government will spend your money on the experts to tell you how to eat healthy, but they have no control over the lobbyists.

There will be commercials and information telling you high fructose corn syrup is from corn and is good for you, that sugary cereals are energy for you, and that diets are the answer. Just keep in mind those who tell you this are also making money from you. Beware.

What If I Can't Always Make Smart Choices?

We would all like to make smart choices all the time, but what if you are really hungry, and your environment doesn't offer healthful food? What should you do? If you can't find foods that are high in nutritional value and you are hungry, choose a balanced portion and then make up for it later when you have an opportunity to make healthier choices.

Let's take, for example, a parent at the ball park with the kids. Everyone is hungry and it could be four hours before the next meal. What do you do? A hot dog on white bread may not be the healthiest choice, but perhaps, given your situation, it may be the smartest choice, in comparison with the chicken wings, fried onion rings or fries. Let's suppose you never eat hotdogs because of the nitrates, food coloring, antibiotics, preservatives and the fact that, by most peoples' standards, you have turned into a food snob. The problem is, if you wait eight hours to eat, you could be in worse trouble. You have to decide which is the lesser evil.

If you eat fruit and include a small tropical drink, trying to stay healthy and forgoing balance, in less than two hours, you will be exhausted, cranky, wishing you could go home and starving for a big meal. So much for a day at the ball park with the kids! The smart choice would be the hot dog, maybe only part of the bun, and a piece of fruit. Forget the tropical drink. There isn't enough protein or fiber to offset the high calories of sugar.

The hot dog isn't the healthiest choice, but for the situation you're in, it is the smartest. I suppose you could come fully equipped with a lunch box with perfectly balanced healthy food. I applaud those who are organized and dedicated enough to do that. Although I have great intentions, I am never quite able to. No, I'm the parent with the screaming kids, challenged enough with finding seats, and not losing a child in the process.

If you make smart choices at the ball park, you will come home thinking clearly and not like a ravenous beast eating anything in sight.

Energy Without Calories: a Disastrous Combination.

We live in a society that wants the energy without the calories. If there is a product that provides that, then we believe that we have beaten the system. The marketplace provides energy products without the calories, but what you are tapping into is your nervous system. There are stimulants that produce nervous energy. Nervous energy comes at a price! Every time you take a stimulant, you inhibit your body's own ability to produce energy and you become dependant on the stimulant, such as caffeine, or other products on the market, those so-called *natural* energy stimulants.

Every time you tap into your nervous system for energy, you zap your adrenal glands. These glands release hormones that give your body a short term burst of energy. These glands help you survive by using a flight *or fight* syndrome. In other words, the hormones they secrete are designed to give you a burst of energy when food isn't available, and it becomes necessary for your survival enabling you to run from a predator, or stay and fight.

Once the hormones are finished circulating through your system, you become tired, and develop a huge craving for starchy, sugary foods which is how the body calms the circulating hormones. The problem is that once you eat the sugar to relieve the effect of the hormonal stress, the added sugar triggers an insulin reaction, which causes further fatigue, and the motivation to take a stim-

184 | Six Steps to Never Diet Again

ulant to regain your energy becomes overwhelming. This happens when someone drinks coffee all day long or has the need to drink caffeinated beverages just to feel good again.

Stimulants Give a Short-Term Boost That Causes Long-Term Problems

What they don't know is that abusive use of these stimulants combined with a poor diet can cause adrenal exhaustion. The adrenal glands become tired from the constant surge of these hormones, combined with poor diet choices. Adrenal exhaustion comes in different levels. Some people have such a low level, they are unable to function until they've had their stimulant fix, while others experience fatigue only some of the time. Over the long haul, this energy use can lead to a more chronic state of exhaustion, which results in depression, chronic fatigue, weight gain (especially in the midsection), a feeling of brain fog, dizziness, and light headedness.

Through the years, I have seen how stimulants have given some people this false sense of energy, enabling them to be more physically and mentally productive. Before a workout, they take the stimulant, and upon completion, they resort to additional stimulants to keep them going. Initially, they lose considerable amounts of weight and are very hyper on very few calories. They are high on energy and look and feel thin at the same time. This can be addictive, but also extremely dangerous. Eventually, this cycle can result in chronic fatigue, which is very difficult to recover from. It can start with one or two diet drinks with caffeine and then lead to an all-day indulgence. This can then lead to further experimentation of herbs and other over-the-counter stimulants.

Unfortunately, I have witnessed this abuse within my 30 years of training people. I have seen how individuals take this artificial energy approach, which seems to work for a while. They feel as if it keeps them thin and gives them a lot of energy. These people believe they have fooled their bodies. What they don't realize is that the body is a very smart machine and it will do everything it can to get balanced, including overworking the adrenal glands and stressing out major organs.

Over the years, it results in serious weight gain and exhausting fatigue. A large number of these cases result in more serious health problems, such as fibromyalgia, chronic fatigue, depression, and morbid obesity. It is almost impossible to reason with clients while they are thin and full of nervous artificial energy. It is only years later, when they are suffering from symptoms of abuse, that they are willing to make a change.

It is Possible to Regain Your Natural Energy?

It is a process that can happen following the six-step approach I am advocating. It will also require a more diligent effort to thoroughly ensure proper recovery. There will be foods and supplements that will be specific to your recovery. Once again, the green plant foods tend to be the most healing for all the reasons mentioned and processed low-fiber sugar foods are the most damaging.

Stimulants That Harm

Two cups of coffee or tea are not considered abusive. There is enough research to support moderate consumption of coffee and tea can actually be beneficial. Where you need to be careful is in the consumption of soft drinks with caffeine, sport drinks, or herbal-energy diet aids. When the caffeine is added to give you more energy, eventually your body will forget how to make its own energy, and your adrenal gland will depend on that caffeine or stimulant to get you moving. Before you know it, you are exhausted without it, and your body has become dependant on this outside stimulant.

If the coffee pot is still brewing at 3:00 in the afternoon and it becomes a regular ritual to keep you motivated, or if there are frequent tea and caffeine splurges throughout the day, you need to reevaluate your current energy situation, and realize this is a dead end that leads to obesity and poor health.

At some point, you are going to have to figure out that your body is a machine, and if you don't figure out how to manage it the right way, it will be forced to compensate in harmful ways just to survive.

ELEVEN

COMMUNICATING THROUGH THE MUSCLE

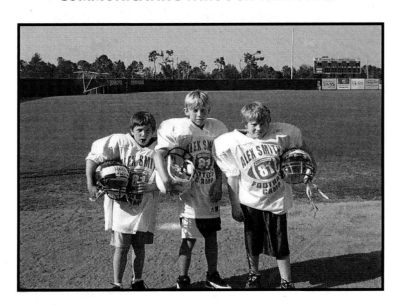

Exercise is Awesome

Exercise makes you better. It is that simple. Exercise is the single most important thing you can do for your body that has the most immediate impact in improving your quality of life. Exercise is the "*on*" switch, the stimulus that enables our bodies to grow stronger, healthier and leaner.

That's nothing new, right? Most of us have heard that exercise is good for us and needs to be part of our lives. The problem is trying to *make* it a part of our lives. Busy schedules and numerous responsibilities seem to take precedence. Finding a half-hour or so to exercise can seem like an impossible task, especially after a long day at work when you have little energy or desire, and all you want to do is sit in front of the television and unwind. You are emotionally and mentally exhausted, which makes you feel physically tired.

Maybe you have lower back or joint pain, and your muscles already ache. You can't imagine how movement could relieve you of your exhaustion. The reality is that some of us are scared to physically exert ourselves, don't have the schedules that permit time to exercise, and/or lack the motivation to exercise. I'm going to show you how you can get all the benefits of exercise without any of your reality getting in the way.

Internal Benefits From Muscle Movement

As muscles are physically exerted, they send electrical messages to every cell, demanding the entire body to live up to the challenge that has been asked of them. It is as if the whole body is put on alert. Moving muscles starts a chain reaction that makes the entire body perform at a significantly higher level. The results are amazing. The body becomes stronger from the inside out.

Communicating Through the Muscle

Muscle movement is the single most dramatic impact you can make on your body. When we move muscles, it is as if we turn switches on inside of our cells. It is the difference between turning your body *on* or *off*. A study done with non-exercisers found that just 10 minutes a day of muscle movement resulted in significant health improvements for the subjects tested. Perhaps because just 10 minutes a day can be the difference between turning *on* or *off* the switch for good health.

Exercise Makes the Body Grow Stronger and Healthier in the Most Amazing Ways:

1. Increases the number of capillaries that their ability to deliver oxygen deep inside muscles.

2. Red blood cells ability to carry more oxygen.

3. Blood flows more easily through the artery walls which improves blood pressure.

4. Increases the strength of your heart, enabling it to pump more blood to the rest of the body.

5. Increases the amount of oxygen your lungs can take to the rest of the body.

6. Increases the size and number of energy units (called mitochondria) inside the cells. The more mitochondria, the more energy for the cell.

7. Hormones work more efficiently.

8. Improves muscular strength. Lack of exercise causes our muscles to atrophy, and stimulating our muscles causes growth.

9. Improves bone density.

10. Enzyme activity increases. Enzymes serve as the spark that enables the cells to perform.

11. Fat burning increases.

12. Brain function improves, enabling us to think more clearly and achieve happier moods.

What Makes Muscle Movement so Powerful

Excercize is the only language our body understands. It is the only form of communication you have with your body. It would be wonderful if we could verbally demand our bodies to grow strong and healthy. You cannot command your body to improve muscle tone or improve your immunity. You can think it, you can wish it, but the body will not respond until you move it. Exercise causes physical changes to occur, not just the obvious muscle toning that looks great in a pair of jeans, but the internal changes you may not be aware of. Exercise turns a switch *"on"* that causes all bodily functions to improve.

A Sedentary Life Tells The Body to Decay

Living a sedentary life turns an internal switch *"off."* If you don't communicate with your body by moving muscles, it is told to decay. It is as if you're telling your body it isn't needed. As your body decays internally, muscles begin to atrophy (which means you lose muscle tissue). As muscles become soft from inactivity, they marble with fat. Marbled fatty muscle tissue slows down the metabolism. A slow metabolism causes an increase in extra body fat, which makes you an incubator for toxins. The more toxic you become, the more vulnerable you are for serious illness.

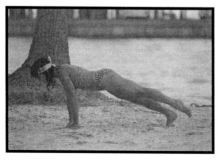

Myrna's beach plank

Muscles That Aren't Needed Go Away

It is only through muscles that you can alter your entire physical wellbeing. Diet supports and enables the process, but it is the muscle tissue that uses the nutrients to trigger a cascade of positive events. It is the muscles that command your body to be healthy. Fat does nothing but hang around. Muscle is what drives the bus. The more muscle tissue you have and the healthier you maintain it, the more capacity you have to be healthier. The body wants you to make it strong.

We Don't Live in a Perfect World

In a perfect world you would dedicate 45 minutes a day to exercise, knowing it is the most worthwhile investment you're making in your health. Our bodies want 45 minutes to one hour of prescribed exercise per day. The type of exercise that makes your heart pump, muscles contract, and leaves you totally drenched in sweat! The reality for most of us is that our schedules don't permit this, and even if they did, we would never last more than 10 minutes. We may not enjoy sweating profusely, having our heart pump wildly and muscles burn.

The problem is that the human body was designed to move vigorously. The heart and muscles improve the more we push them. Exercise keeps us balanced and makes us grow stronger. So what do you do when there is no time to exercise, and you're not even sure you have the strength to do it anyway?

The first solution is to figure out how to move muscles to turn switches *"on"* that trigger your body into a state of growth instead of decay. Since your life is already busy, you have to figure out how to do this without too much inconvenience in your daily routine. This isn't the best solution…just the first solution.

Challenging muscles to move is not exclusive to an exercise program. Muscles don't care if you are in a gym, your living room, at work, or grocery shopping. To the body, it is all the same. Muscles want to be challenged. Remember that this is the message that tells them to improve, so if you don't have time to exercise, you'll have to figure out how to challenge muscles within your daily routine.

Most people avoid exerting themselves past their comfort zone. It is only when muscles are pushed beyond what is comfortable that they're forced to be better than before. As the muscles improve, everything else does too! The whole body steps up to meet the muscles' cry to become better. If your reality does not make even 15 minutes a day of exercise possible, I'm still going to show you how to turn the switch "on" for growth, strength and good health within your day.

Muscles Are Fresh Even if You're Not

Let's face it. A long day at work can really make you feel wiped out. The truth is, unless you have a very physical job where you are walking several miles, it is unlikely that you are physically tired. You might be emotionally or mentally exhausted, which makes you feel physically tired, but your muscles are not.

Exercise can relieve you of your mental and emotional exhaustion. It sounds crazy, but this is exactly what exercise does. It takes about 10 minutes of movement before your grumpy, tired self wears off. When you exercise, you cause a chemical reaction. This chemical reaction affects your immune system, muscular and skeletal system, hormone and nervous system. There is not one cell in your body that doesn't heed the call to improve, to grow, to make you better.

Methods Of Movements That Will Totally Change Your Life

1. *Healthy Fit:* Moving Muscle in Everyday Movement

2. *Athletic Fit:* Moving Muscle Purposefully for a Designated Time

1. Healthy Fit

Turning Switches on in Your Daily Routine

Our daily routine is usually done through comfortable, leisurely physical movements. We seldom push our muscles to work harder as we move through our day, which is exactly what is needed to make the muscle stronger and improve our health. The good news is that it only takes 10-15 seconds of vigorous challenging movement to bring about a change for most people.

A healthy, fit lifestyle is for everyone, but for those who are unable to find the time or motivation to exercise, being *Healthy Fit* becomes critical. Exercise communicates to our body that we want to stay alive; we want to grow in strength and health. A *Healthy Fit* lifestyle allows for us to communicate within our everyday routines. Here is how and why this works. Your body lives for the moment. It reacts to immediate stimulus, which serves us well when trying to be *Healthy Fit*. Let me show you how the living-for-the-moment concept can be used optimally in a Healthy *Fit* lifestyle.

Being Healthy Fit

Being healthy fit is a function of stimulating the muscles with small burst of intensity throughout the day. It is as if you turn up the volume in your everyday movement. Walking from your car to the store moves muscles but if you walk at a very fast pace, at a point where you literally can feel your legs tingle, then you will have worked the muscle just enough to send a message to the brain that causes a positive reaction throughout your body. Do this 10-15 times in your normal routine, and it can add up to 30 minutes at the gym. At first it will seem a little strange, but you will find that there are at least 15-20 times during the day that you will have opportunities, lasting 30 seconds to 2 minutes, to move vigorously within your daily routine. All it really takes is just 10-15 seconds of a muscle burn to ignite a positive change in your body.

Take Lisa, who is a new mom. She gets at least 10-15 minutes throughout the day of some great arm-firming exercises lifting her son of 15 pounds. She purposely does some variations in lifting and swinging the baby that she swears have made a difference. With both of my children, I can remember taking several minutes throughout the day performing these same lifts. The children loved it and so did my arms.

Think of how many places you walk to and from your vehicle. Can you walk vigorously to create a slight burst of intensity? Try quickly running up stairs or taking two stairs at a time. After 15 seconds of these, even top athletes can feel the tingle in their legs. When you go to the grocery store for a few items, evenly distribute the groceries among both arms and do small bicep curls until you reach your car. When you find yourself standing in line as when you go to the grocery store, try holding your stomach in as tight as you can, pulling your belly button towards your spine, and at the same time squeeze your buttocks muscles. After 1-2 minutes of this, you will feel your muscles burn. When at work, I can find periodic opportunities to squeeze and flex all day long.

> *Seize every opportunity to move throughout your day, and make it as vigorous as you can. Muscles have to be continually reminded that they are needed, or they go away, and what you get instead is fat.*

My son is involved in Little League. Most parents bring chairs and sit and watch while their children run around. This is great for the kids, not so good for their folks. There is an apparatus you can buy that attaches to the back wheel of a road bike. It turns a road bike into a stationary bike. You can buy them at most bike shops. Instead of sitting, I bring my bike apparatus, called a bike trainer, and pedal my way through his game. My son doesn't care if I am sitting or moving as long as my eyes are on him. What a great way for both of us to get exercise!

How about a few leg squats while you prepare dinner? Works great while you chop, grind or mix. Of course, your family will think you're crazy, but do you really care?

These are all great examples of 10-15 second blasts, that if done enough throughout your day can make a significant improvement in your body. I have found any amount is good, but at least 15 blasts of 30-second to one-minute muscle intensity movements throughout your normal routine, **can and will** improve your body.

Athletes Are Made Not Born

As soon as you start setting goals and move your body towards reaching those goals, you are an athlete. Athletes don't start with muscular, lean bodies; they start with a goal and a plan. Lance Armstrong was no less of an athlete after cancer treatment than when he won the tour five times! The only difference between walking around the block after cancer treatment and winning the Tour-de-France, one of the most grueling athletic feats in cycling, is the muscle work and adaptation process that is required to reach both goals. Both required setting goals and building and adapting muscles, one was walking around the block and the other involved 100-mile bike ride through the mountains. Athletes set goals and move a little bit every day towards reaching them. There is no difference between the athlete who is 100 pounds overweight setting daily 10-15 minute movement goals or a World Class cyclist. Both are setting goals and working towards achieving them.

"Being an athlete is something you choose, not something you are born with."

2. Athletic Fit

Being Athletic Fit is Choosing to be an Athlete

Taking it to the next level is what distinguishes being Healthy Fit from being Athletic Fit. The Athletic Fit lifestyle takes a more deliberate approach, setting goals and using systems of measurement to achieve those goals. You begin to measure your performance and set goals weekly or monthly to improve. Instead of walking 10-15 minutes, you set a goal to walk 25-30 minutes, as well as setting goals to walk the same distance in less time.

Going out for a leisurely walk is great if you want to get some fresh air. A leisure walk doesn't send the same message as a muscle-challenging walk. As you pump your arms and get your legs moving, you can feel your thighs, calves and butt muscles working. As you feel your muscles working, you have turned the internal switch on which results in more bone density, increased circulation, lower blood pressure, a stronger heart, stronger muscles, more fat burning, more cell energy, better skin, hair, brain and mood.

As soon as you set goals such as deciding you will increase your walking distance a few more minutes every week or time yourself for each mile, you have crossed over into true athlete status. Athletes measure their performance and strive to improve. You can be an athlete with any muscle movement at any level. Every coach has his or her own method for training athletes, but regardless of the methodology, it basically comes down to three basic principles:

THREE BASIC TRAINING PRINCIPLES FOR ATHLETES

1. *Build A Foundation:* Base training - Building strength in the muscles and heart, slowly and comfortably

2. *Muscle Specificity:* Pushing certain groups of muscles for an intended purpose

3. *Muscle Balance:* Not allowing specifically trained muscles to over-power weaker ones

Athletic training is when you set goals and monitor your performance within these three basic principles. It is no more complicated than that. Over a period of time, if these three principles are done properly, you're an awesome athlete with one heck of a body!

1. Building a Foundation

All Athletes Build a Foundation

As muscles build and adapt to a workload, they begin to build a foundation. This foundation is usually referred to as **base training**. You can't work muscle intensely until you have a solid foundation. Base training prepares the muscle, tendons, and connective tissue for the workload. **Base training is _consistent, comfortable_ and _repetitive_ muscle work.** It should not be too uncomfortable. You have to prepare the muscle to be pushed. In other words you have to prepare your muscles to be fit before you can be fit. It helps if you have been doing muscle work in your daily routine, as I explained with being Healthy Fit. There is still nothing however that prepares you for continuous, repetitive muscle work better than just actually doing it!

How to Build a Muscle Foundation

Building a solid muscle foundation can take months, even years. But unless you have a solid base, exercise can cause injury. Muscles cannot be pushed before they are ready. If you are doing an exercise program now that isn't much fun and you feel is too difficult, then there is a good chance you haven't spent enough time in base training. Exercise intensity, the profuse sweating, heart-beating, muscle-burning vigorous work is fun only if you are doing it after a base training period. It is only after you have prepared your body with a solid base training that hitting the muscles with bursts of intensity for prolonged periods actually feels good!

When you get to this point, your muscle-to-fat ratio has changed, and your body is much better at burning fat than storing it. You will find you are able to exercise at higher intensities without feeling tired. In fact, your perceived exertion changes, and you can do a lot of intense exercise without feeling as if you exercised hard!

If You Are Unfit and Overweight, Base Training is Easy

The less fit and more overweight you are, the easier your base training should be, focusing on less exercise more often. In the beginning, base training is properly done when you exercise throughout the day, maybe 10 minutes in the morning, 5 minutes at lunch and 10 minutes at night. Once your muscles get stronger, try 15 minutes in the morning and 10 minutes at night. After a month or two, work up to 25-30 minutes at one time.

Once your muscles are strong enough to work up to 25-30 minutes at one time, you can tap into the added benefit of heart rate work and fat burning, which occurs with continuous movement over a prolonged period. It is true that with both Healthy Fit and Athletic Fit work, muscles turn switches on, but the difference with Athletic Fit activity is that the longer periods of exercise take you to a higher level. It is like turning the dimmer switch on high.

Building a Foundation

When building a foundation, don't worry about intensity; work towards building longer periods of continuous movement. You must first build muscle tolerance before you think about what your heart is doing or how hard you work your muscles.

Athletes Work Their Hearts

Becoming an athlete involves training the heart. It is part of the natural process of becoming more physically fit. Working the heart muscle requires heat rate training which is measured through the number of beats your heart pumps per minute. Based on the number of heart beats per minute, you can measure your physical performance. Whether it is a leaner body or a certain gain in fitness, working the heart muscle accelerates the physical changes that occur with exercise. This stimulates the body to create endorphins, feel good chemicals that circulate your bloodstream after a good heart-pumping, muscle-driving workout.

You should do heart-rate training over a period of time, somewhere in the range of 20-45 minutes, continuously, without stopping. If you have developed a solid muscle foundation, this should be fairly easy. There is actually a **Target Heart Rate** range where all this cool stuff starts happening. It is in this heart rate range where you want to exercise for 20-45 minutes. If you exercise below this range, it is still better than not exercising at all, but it won't create the same enzymes that are responsible for burning body fat and kicking your body to a higher level, creating feel good hormones.

Having said that, you need to remember that first-timers in base training, working the heart below the target range, could be the perfect level to prepare the muscles. Exercising at the lower end of their target heart rate range allows beginners to slowly and safely progress. I don't recommend pushing your heart rate at maximum levels until you have completed a base training program for several months. Keep in mind that the muscles allow the heart to work for prolonged periods. You need to make sure they are ready.

How to Figure Out Target Heart Rate

Target heart rate is the target range you're aiming for good health. It is based on your age. The older you are, the lower your heart rate needs to be to get the same effect as younger people who can push their hearts harder.

Target Heart Rate (THR) Formula

220 – Age = _____ Maximum Heart Rate (MHR)

MHR _____ X (65%-85%) = _____ (THR)

---

220 minus your age is your maximum heart rate (MHR), that is if you are really pushing it, you may last 10-15 seconds at this level if you are really fit and have years of base training. You don't want to push that hard unless you have years of muscle preparedness. The desired range is the Target Heart Rate (THR). This happens when you work your heart 65%-85% of your maximum rate. If your muscles are less fit, it is best to stay closer to the 65% range. If you are a seasoned athlete with years of base training, then it will feel more comfortable at the higher range.

The key with target heart rate training is to stay consistent and work towards longer durations. This type of training is called aerobic training.

Aerobic Exercise

When you work your body aerobically (within your target range) for longer periods of time, at least 20 minutes, the body creates enzymes that increase fat burning while becoming more efficient at delivering oxygen to the muscles. This type of training results in a strong circulatory and respiratory system, which means it increases blood volume, lowers blood pressure, creates good cholesterols, and increases the amount of oxygen the lungs can absorb and distribute to all of your cells.

How To Count Your Heart Beats Per Minute

Find your pulse on your wrist. Use your fingers, not your thumb to count. Look at a watch to count for six seconds the number of beats you feel. Start with number one and round up for half beats. Add a zero to the number of beats you count for six seconds this will give you an approximation of the number of beats per minute.

Example:

If for six seconds you count 11 ½ beats. Round up a beat and add a zero. The target heart rate would be 120 beats per minute.

If I'm Overweight How Hard Should I Push My Heart?

If you are in good condition, because you exercise regularly, but carry around an extra 20-30 pounds because you haven't figured out how to eat right, then the same rules apply to you that apply to anyone else. The only difference is that the same movement will be a lot harder for you to do, and you will end up having to modify your intensity level.

Not all heart rates are the same. The THR formula is just an average calculation. Fifteen percent of the population at either end will not fall within the normal curve. Also, medications that slow down the heart rate make this formula irrelevant. The best method will always be how you feel.

If you are overweight and out of shape, once again the same rules still apply. The big difference for you will be that your heart will be working very hard without you realizing it. When your heart is **not in good condition and you're overweight,** your heart will beat much faster than someone whose heart is in good shape. An out-of –shape overweight person doesn't look as if they are working that hard. They don't sweat or move vigorously, and yet, internally they may be working very hard. It is the opposite of what it appears.

You can see the evidence of this when one of these overweight, out-of-shape people goes for a walk, and their heart rate climbs past a comfortable range. They haven't done all that much, yet a conditioned person may have to jog at a fairly strong pace to get a similar heart rate. The overweight, unconditioned person may be working harder than the jogger who is pushing a fast pace. The outer appearance shows an out-of-shape person barely sweating with a high heart rate, and an athlete drenched with sweat moving vigorously with a lower heart rate. The out-of-condition heart is working much harder than the sweaty athlete's.

When you are out of shape, you haven't developed the internal equipment that enables you to move vigorously, like the increased enzymes, energy units in the cell, blood volume and muscle fiber. **This is why I recommend that you start exercising comfortably, and focus on building muscle strength and endurance, not intensity.** Heart rate training is less important than moving muscles comfortably for a longer duration of time. Your best measurement of performance is perceived exertion.

Perceived Exertion

Don't get too caught up in what your heart is doing. The real key will always be your perceived exertion, which is how you feel. You want to keep your perceived exertion at about a level 5 or 6 (1 being easy and 10 being hard). Exercising at a lower heart rate means there is less chance for injury and more probability you will spend more time moving, which is exactly what you need when trying to build-up muscle tolerance.

When you are focused on your base training, the emphasis is more on muscle preparedness and less on heart rate training. Perceived exertion should always be the number one measurement when exercising. Even when you are working at your target heart rate, you want a perceived exertion of a level 5-7, which falls in the range of 65%-85% of your maximum heart rate. Training your heart to work at a certain rate for a period of time, such as recommended at your target rate of 65%-85%, makes a huge difference in your body's ability to burn fat and deliver oxygen. Target heart rate training works even more muscles than just the muscle pump you get from working isolated muscles. No matter what type of exercise or intensity, perceived exertion is the number one indicator you should use to know how much is appropriate.

As you become more fit, you will be able to push your muscles and heart much harder without feeling as if you are working that hard. In other words, your perceived exertion changes the more conditioned you are. Keep in mind, if you work too far beyond what feels good, you will not be able to work beyond what does good. A good rule of thumb is to keep your perceived exertion between level 5-7.

Perceived Exertion Chart

1	2	3	4	5	6	7	8	9	10
Very Easy		Easy		Medium		Medium Hard			Very Hard

BELOW 50%   **65%-85%**   **ABOVE 85%**

Percentage Heart Rate

What Happens to my Body at Maximum Heart Rate?

Higher heart rates usually mean sore muscles. High heart rate is a result of pushing the upper end of your performance which can be just what is needed to reach higher levels of fitness for the experienced athlete. This is not a good idea if you don't have a solid base. Unless your muscles are ready for this type of training, you could get injured.

High-End Anaerobic Training

Experienced athletes work their heart rate percentage higher than 80% of their target range when they are looking to improve their fitness levels. This is called **anaerobic training**. It is the opposite of aerobic training. It works directly from the muscle, and it is more about brute strength than moving oxygen around. Experienced athletes do this type of training when they are looking to get that extra hardness in the muscle. They are hoping the added strength will give them that extra edge.

Lactic acid is produced when muscles are challenged. *Muscles love to be challenged, but if they have been allowed to be sedentary for a period of time, they have forgotten how to be pushed. It won't take much for lactic acid to build up. Lactic acid is an acid that is produced in the muscle when it has been worked beyond its strength capability. It is a sure way to make you stop moving before you hurt yourself. Lactic acid isn't serious. It just makes your muscles sore and stiff. In a few days the body cleans it out of the muscle. The more conditioned the muscle, the less you will experience lactic acid build up.*

This type of training is most effective in improving strength and results in a more defined muscle. It is what most people call *"buffed."* They do this type of heart rate training in spikes, with small burst of intensity followed by lower levels of aerobic exercise. Since it is done in intervals, it is called **interval training**. This type of exercise places the highest workload on muscles. If you are fit enough to do this type of exercise training, your muscles will get more muscular. The more muscular you are, the less fat you have, and the higher your metabolism. Once again, interval training is great only if you have a really good foundation. Otherwise, you risk burnout and injury.

How to Do Intervals

If you are going to push the intensity, make sure you warm-up a minimum of 20-30 minutes at the lower end of your target heart rate range before you push your muscles hard. With interval training, just a few spikes in the middle of your workout can be enough to increase your level of fitness. I have a rule of thumb of just 3-5 intervals of all out intensity is usually enough of a catalyst to bump you to a higher fitness level. If you can do more than 5 intervals, then chances are you really aren't pushing hard enough during the interval. The rest periods in between the intervals should be at least twice as long as the interval.

Example of Interval Training Workout:

Warm up (20-30 minutes)
at Target Heart Rate (60%-75%)

Interval Training (15 minutes)
1 minute hard – 80%-95%;
2 minutes target range – 60%-75%

(repeat Interval Training 5 times)

Cool Down (10 minutes)
at Target Heart Rate (60%-75%)

Base Training is About Building up Muscle Tolerance

People always ask me how they will know when they are ready for more. One way to know you are ready for more is when the same routine that gave you spectacular results initially, doesn't seem to give you the same results. In fact, you are very comfortable with your routine and can't understand why you are feeling fatter.

Does this mean that exercise doesn't work anymore? NO.... What this means is that you are in better condition. The same amount of exercise doesn't present a challenge to you anymore. **Your body has become very comfortable with your routine, so the body has adapted to movement that was once difficult. To get the same results as when you first started, you have to challenge the muscles once more.** The good news is, because you have built a muscle foundation, you will be able to take on more. This is what moves you to the next level of fitness, and once again, the body begins to change. Fitness is a function of how well you adapt to specific work loads. What once was very challenging could seem very easy a year later.

Athletes Do Strength Training

Strength training is defined as pushing muscles beyond their comfort zone, for designated periods of time, for the purpose of making them stronger.

When you push muscles beyond their comfort threshold, it triggers a response from the body to make improvements in order to adapt to the work load you have requested. This results in a stronger and healthier you. If you do this type of muscle work and adaptation on a regular basis, it is referred to as **strength training**.

There are many different ways to develop strength. You can use resistance by adding weights, as in weight training with dumbbells, or use the weight of your own body, in sit-ups and push-ups. Pushing muscles past their comfort zone forces them to adapt to be stronger. It is in this adaptation process that the entire body becomes better.

2. Muscle Specificity
Athletic Fit Works Muscle Specificity

Let's say you set an athletic goal and you're diligently training to do your first 6-mile run. Or, you signed up for a 3-day, 60-mile walk. Whatever your goal, there is a good chance you will work specific muscles over and over again with the same pattern of movement to reach your goal. This is called **muscle specificity**. It means that you are specifically working certain groups of muscles for an intended purpose. The more muscle specific you become, the more attention you will need to pay to **muscle balance**. If you continuously work specific muscles and not work all your muscles equally, the over-trained muscle will cause an imbalance, which will cause injury, such as muscle pulls, strains and tendonitis. Muscle imbalances occur when stronger muscles overpower weaker ones. A lot of people think they can just stretch out tired muscles or include more rest periods between workouts. Although this is all good, it is not muscle balance, and you can still get injured. This is why athletes cross train to avoid over-training certain muscles.

3. Muscle Balance
Muscle Balance Prevents Injuries

Muscle balance means strengthening the opposite muscles of the specific muscles you are training. If your goal is to run a 6-mile event, the muscles in the back lower leg (calf muscle or gastrocniumus) will be worked much harder in comparison to the muscles in the front of the lower leg, (tibialis anterior);. Therefore, you need to do toe lifts to work the front anterior muscle that lays over your shin bone and is directly opposite of the calf muscle in the back of your leg.

An injury that frequently occurs because of muscle imbalance is *shin splints*. The calf muscle (gastrocnemius) overpowers the shin muscle (tibalous), which causes a tear along the shin bone. Walking would be a good cross training for running because walking works the front shin muscle, whereas running emphasizes the back of the lower leg. Cycling over-trains the muscles in the hip area as well as the front of the upper thigh. A few workouts a week in the pool swimming or using a kick board would help strengthen the opposite muscles by working the butt muscle and hamstring in the opposite way they are worked on a bike.

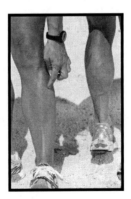

When Muscle Injuries Occur

Most injuries occur when muscles are not prepared for higher levels of intensity and or when stronger muscles overpower weaker ones. Almost always, weaker muscles will be on the opposite side of overworked muscles. If you contract one muscle all the time, the muscle that sits on the opposite side will be weaker. It is the weaker muscle you need to strengthen.

Athletic training isn't the only activity that causes this either. Everyday movement can overwork certain muscles more than others, causing an imbalance that leads to chronic back, shoulder and neck pain. Just standing all day at your job can cause the lower back muscles to overpower the abdominal muscles. To properly balance the back muscles, you would work the weaker abdominal muscles. This would eliminate lower back pain. If you bend down over a computer all day, the neck and back of the shoulders are worked more than the front of the body. Muscle balance could be achieved by strengthening the chest to counter the imbalance created in crouching over your computer all day.

Another reason for injuries is when muscles are improperly prepared for higher levels of intensity, or do not have enough time to recover from hard work. Muscle preparedness and proper recovery is about understanding base training, which is knowing when to work the muscles at a comfortable level.

All Athletes Come Back to Base Training

Base training is not just where you start, it is where all seasoned athletes return to as part of their continued work out regimen. The comfortable, easy muscle work in base training serves as a good recovery for fit athletes. Even elite athletes spend 50% of their fitness hours in base training and the other time working hard. How well you recover from your hard day determines your fitness level. Exercise won't work unless you recover from it.

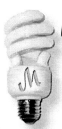

Recovery
It is in the recovery process where the body repairs and makes muscles stronger. So, you should work hard only 50% of the time and easy the rest of the time.

Building Base

1. **Prepare Muscles**
   a. Strengthen all muscles equally
   b. Work muscles less intense more often

2. **Set Goals to Move for a Specific Amount of Time.**
   a. Work up to 30 minutes at one time.
   b. Work up to 30 minutes at target heart rate.
   c. Include burst of vigorous intensity in the middle of target heart rate workout.

Daily Example

15-minute muscle builder routine. Work up to 3-5 sets of each. Each set is between 12-15 repetitions Take as much rest needed between sets

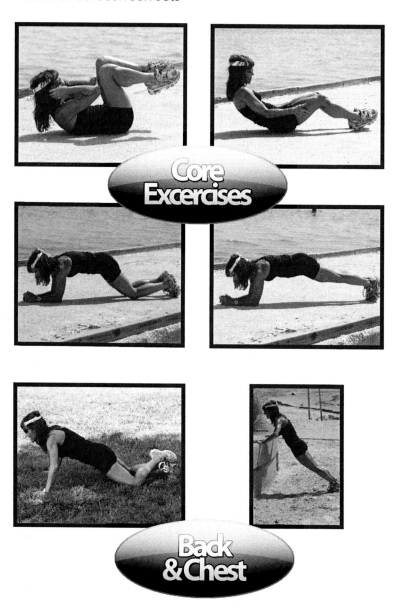

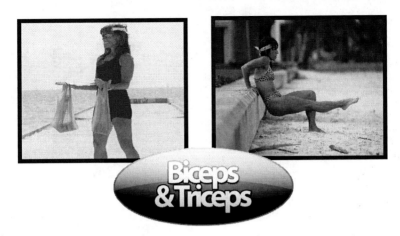

Biceps & Triceps

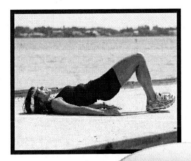
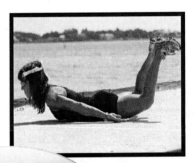

Buttocks

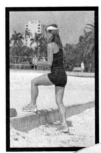
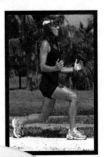

Hamstrings & Quadriceps

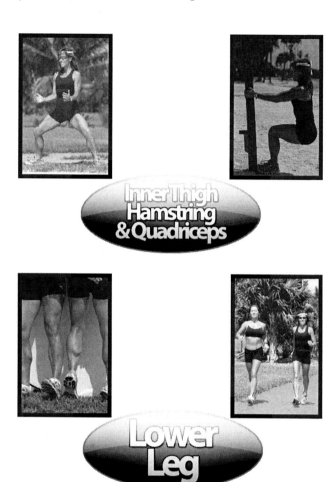

TWELVE

EMPOWERMENT

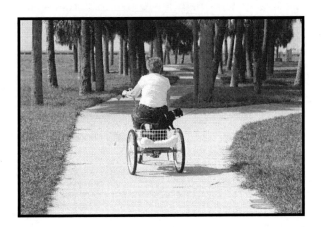

Rubber Hits the Road

This is the part where the rubber hits the road. At this point, you have a lot of information. Will you be able to make it work for you? How are you going to make yourself do this stuff? What is going to empower you to be successful?

Empowerment is a big subject. If you go to the library or your favorite bookstore, you will find shelves of self-help books on empowerment. If that doesn't help, there are coaches, trainers, physiologists, ministers, motivational speakers, and best friends. All good stuff, but it won't work unless you have become honest about yourself first.

Before you can work on empowerment, you have to **Get Real!** To Get Real means removing the veil, and coming out of denial. Take a hard look at yourself and what's going on around you. If you live in denial, you believe and say things that aren't real, and you stop believing. What I mean by this is that you stop believing in yourself, and you sell yourself short.

I suppose it is much healthier to live in denial than to become depressed, feel hopeless, and lose your self esteem. People do this denial thing because they don't have a way out, and it saves them from total self-destruction. The problem is unless you come clean and get totally real with yourself, you can't overcome what is causing you to be in denial.

Denial is when you claim you can't exercise because of some external influence, like the weather is always bad, or you have poor heredity that doesn't allow you to move, or you don't need to exercise. You have a slow metabolism that makes you fat is another excuse you may use. Your stressful life causes you to overeat, you believe. If you are in denial, you don't need to be empowered, because your situation is not your fault. You are a victim; therefore, your choices are justified. This is great for your self preservation, but you won't solve anything until you take an honest look at yourself and realize this is about you and how <u>you take on this challenge</u>. Being a victim will only get in the way of your success.

To become empowered, you must first be self aware. You have to admit there are things about yourself that you know are making it difficult to be empowered. Trying to be honest with yourself can be the hardest part. It is so much easier to be a legend in your own mind. Everyone who has gone through the six-step process will tell you it works like magic, but only after a point of self awareness.

Your challenges may never fully disappear, but what a difference it makes when you are empowered to deal with them. The more you empower yourself, the less they surface.

Me, Myself - and You!

A get real moment for me is wedding cake. Wedding cakes are made from the real stuff, not a packaged mix. Let's face it; people spend some big bucks on wedding cake. I start thinking how good that cake will taste during the church ceremony. When the cake is finally passed out to the guests, I end up eating someone else's piece as well as my own I'm totally aware of my wedding cake problem. I try to empower myself by making sure I don't go to the wedding hungry or in an unbalanced state. I make sure I don't drink too much wine in the beginning and eat plenty of protein in the reception banquet line. I'm fully aware I have some issues, and I have to empower myself before the wedding. If I wasn't honest with myself I would justify the two pieces of cake splurge with the exercise class I did the day before. I would also use the most frequent denial statements of all time… "They are going to throw away expensive cake unless I eat it!" This is an example of denial, and if you are in denial, it takes getting real with yourself before you can move on to empowerment.

I'm Ready to Empower Myself

Perhaps empowerment should be the first step to the six-step process. I didn't want to appear as a muscular cheerleader with a diet book telling you, "Just look at me… you can do it!" Hopefully, by the time you get to this point, you will realize that this is not a diet book! Food issues and being overweight have a lot to do with the fact that once you get into trouble, your body takes over, and it doesn't matter how empowered you are; you are going down! This book is about how to stay out of trouble, so empowerment will work for you.

The best advice on empowerment is that no one will ever be an expert on how to empower you, more than you! If you find something that works, stick with it. If nothing's ever worked, the remaining chapters will offer a few suggestions and guidelines that may help you.

THE FOUR POWERS OF EMPOWERED PEOPLE

1. Power of Suggestion
2. Power of Behavior
3. Power of Association
4. Power of Faith

---

1. Power of Suggestion

The power of suggestion is what you tell your brain. It is your inner voice. It is the language we use when we talk to ourselves. Our inner voice starts with a spark of thought, an idea of what it might be like to be this lean, energetic, healthy person. The spark of thought is pure. It is an idea, a vision. The brain has no way of knowing if thoughts are true or not true. All thoughts enter the brain pure, free of judgment. It isn't until we take that pure thought and run it through our beliefs and personal experiences that the spark of thought can get smothered out quickly.

Our actions become a reflection of our thoughts. It is that simple! We become what we think. If you have been around people who have told you that you are incapable of doing something and if past experiences have been failures, your brain uses this negative language to decide if your suggestions seem possible.

The brain is the main control system, AND it acts according to what it is told. If there are no past experiences or beliefs that tell it otherwise, it believes thoughts, and actually begins to behave based on the thoughts it is given. This is evident with young children who have few past experiences to evaluate their thoughts. Until they form their own belief systems, they will believe what you tell them, and act accordingly.

The term frequently used is *the power of suggestion,* and you can use this power for yourself. The Power of suggestion is ignited through affirmations. Short phrases you tell your brain can be powerful like saying the following: *I am athletic and strong. I am smart and capable. I have a lean energetic body. I live a healthy life that keeps me lean.* Your belief system (past experiences and negative language) may not allow you to believe this is true, so don't give it much thought; just say it to your brain. Say it over and over throughout the day, and let it go. Don't focus too much on if it is true or not. Eventually after you do this enough, the brain is tricked. It begins to believe what you are telling it, and you become a reflection of your affirmation.

> *The power of suggestion is what you suggest to your brain, through daily talk, and the brain is tricked into thinking that is who you are, and you begin to have actions that support this belief.*

This sounds like science fiction, something out of a movie, but, as hard as this is to believe, it is a proven technique that really works!

Eventually if you say something long enough, your brain believes it.

You will begin to notice subtle changes that only you can see. But this is exactly part of the process of rewiring yourself. Diets don't work because we haven't changed our brains. We haven't changed what we want, and therefore, a diet will not be a choice of life, but something you do to solve a problem. It doesn't work! You will always be *on again or off again*, and getting fatter every time!

2. Power of Behavior

Our thoughts and actions are connected. We do things we think about; our behavior reflects our thoughts. You don't think one way and then act another way because there is a direct correlation of your thoughts and beliefs to your actions. If you change your thoughts, then your actions also change.

It also works in reverse. If you act a certain way, your thoughts will soon reflect your behavior. They are connected and also interchangeable. For example, the act of smiling makes you feel happy. Doing things for others makes you feel kind. Unselfish actions create unselfish thoughts. Hurtful, abusive behavior is not connected with a person who has kind and unselfish thoughts.

Similar to the power of suggestion, the power of behavior can rewire our brains through the action, especially when our actions become repetitive. Repeat an action enough times, and it becomes a habit. Just as affirmations are commonly repeated with little thought, habits become actions that are done with little thought.

> *Repetition is powerful because it can change who you are, and what you become sometimes without you even realizing it.*

I want to let you in a on the biggest secret from lean fit people. Not one of them is motivated 100 percent of the time. Maybe not even 50 percent of the time are they motivated to exercise or eat right. The biggest secret is that they follow through because it is something that they do. It is a routine, a habit. If I worked-out only when I was motivated, I wouldn't be fit and enjoy a wonderfully fit body. Other athletes tell me success comes from following a scheduled routine, one they don't think about. **Most people believe these individuals succeed because they think about it but the truth is the opposite. They succeed because they don't think about it. It becomes mindless action.**

Early morning workouts are always my favorite. Probably because, when the alarm goes off, I really don't think too much, I just get up and do my normal routine. It's mindless, and maybe I'm still asleep until I get to the gym and realize my exercise routine is over. If I thought about it too much, there would be hundreds of reasons why I shouldn't go. I usually don't have to worry about too many interruptions at 6:00 in the morning. If I waited until later, well, you can guess how easy it would be for me to lose focus.

This method of establishing mindless routine works for a lot of people, and it may work for you. Pick a time where you know you will do it. Don't try to squeeze it in to your hectic day. That never works!

The key to success is __mindless action__ you schedule into your life that eventually becomes a __habit__ that you do __without much thought__.

Behavior changes thoughts, believe me. You will see subtle changes in how you perceive food and how you start looking at yourself. The power of behavior really works. Your healthy actions begin to work on your brain. Anyone who has ever used this approach says the same thing.

3. Power of Association

There is another energy source similar to the *power of suggestion* and the *power of behavior*. It is the power of association. The power of association has to do with the people we hang out with. Our resources may limit our physical environment. We may not be able to choose where we live or where we go to school. This is not the case with our relationship environment, the people we choose to surround us. You have 100 percent control over the people you choose to let into your life. Take a good look around because you become just like the people you surround yourself with. In fact, there is nothing that will define you more than the people you choose as friends.

Those with similar thoughts and actions are attracted to each other. If you consistently associate with a certain group, your acceptance in the group will be based on mutual thoughts and behavior. You will find that you dress alike, agree on similar views, and participate in the same behavior rituals. You become what you associate with; what you associate with becomes your social environment; your social environment affects your thoughts and actions.

The power of association says we have the power to rewire ourselves by changing who we associate with.

In relation to living a healthy lifestyle, empower yourself by associating with people who live the lifestyle you desire. This isn't intended to sound shallow, but if a lean, energetic body is what you desire, then associate with those who have lean energetic bodies. Why try and reinvent the wheel? These people have already figured out the process of what you are trying to emulate. It is so much easier to join the group and become part of the process.

Don't worry about the physical state you are currently in. It is your mind, not your body that determines those you choose to have a relationship with. Joining a health club where you can meet others who live healthy lifestyles is helpful. Many gyms offer only equipment. Try and find a facility that engages members. Living a healthy lifestyle is more about the relationships you build and less about a particular exercise routine.

Exercise coaching groups, associations or clubs, such as Team in Training, a local walking group, or the YMCA, have group programming opportunities that encourage members to build relationships with others in the group. This is a perfect opportunity to change your social environment by associating with people who live the way you want to. This is all part of the rewiring process. It truly works! Sometimes your only motivation to go to exercise class will be the relationships you have built.

> ## *Don't do it alone!*
>
> *Our human nature is that we prefer to run in packs. It goes back to our prehistoric roots. In the cave man days, our chances for survival were much greater when we worked in a group. We formed tribes that worked together for everyone's benefit. One man alone in the wilderness had less chance of survival than a pack. We really haven't changed much. Although, in today's world, we can isolate ourselves and our chance of survival is much greater than a million years ago. It is very plain and simple. We work better in packs, and we are able to accomplish more in a group than we could ever do on our own.*
>
> *For many people, trying to lose weight and keep it off is one of the biggest challenges. If this is also true for you, then especially consider that any big challenges, whether it is weight loss, career, or personal, is less likely to be achieved when you isolate yourself. In other words, don't do it alone! Find the people you want to associate with that have the power to change your life.*

3. Power of Faith

Faith may be the most powerful energy force on the planet. The power of suggestion, behavior and association is dwarfed in comparison to the *power of faith*. Entire cultures and societies have lived and died all in the name of faith.

Faith is everything you hope for. To be hopeful is to wish for a better future. Faith is when you are unwilling to give up on your hopes and beliefs, even when physical evidence shows it is improbable. Many times people empower themselves through their faith, based on hope.

Faith is believing in something even when you don't have hard evidence.

In keeping a healthy lifestyle, you need to have faith that your rituals and behavior will bring you the body you are hopeful for.

The power of faith is sometimes weak when you get discouraged. You feel lost. It can be difficult to find the path of hope. You begin to look at your past and current situations as your score card. The more you focus on your past failures, the less hope you have. The less likely you will be able to conjure up any faith at all!

Rewiring your brain requires seeing yourself in the future and then having faith that this will be you, even when your current situation and past history don't give evidence to the faith you hold.

So don't look at your past. Your past has nothing to do with hope and faith. Faith and hope are all about you and the future. So spend very little time thinking about your past and spend a whole lot of time thinking about your future.

Have you ever noticed that the most positive people live in the moment and see the future? People who are negative dwell on the past and have no hope for the future. That is because faith and hope are positive energy, and that energy revolves around the future. Hope is all about a bright future. Your past can be a reminder of your failures, and it can trap you into dwelling on it.

Is There a Perfect Formula for Empowerment?

There is no real formula for empowerment because it is an internal process. The four powers mentioned summarize the methods other people use. Through my 30 years of helping others with lifestyle change, I have found an amazing process happens after starting with just one of the powers; eventually the other powers naturally follow. This is really good for you, because the more power you have, the higher probability of success.

It takes pulling out all the stops!

THIRTEEN

LIVE THE LIFE YOU WANT

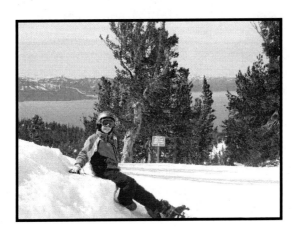

"Live the life you want by using the six steps"

It isn't about the diet, or how much weight you lose. What it really comes down to is: **Can you live the life of the person you want to be?** It isn't about the weight loss, but instead, can you keep it off? Unless you have a plan, once you lose the weight, it will all come back. It has to be **your lifestyle** and **your plan.** Otherwise your life will become a cycle of being on and off a diet.

The six steps will work naturally

You eventually follow a pattern of eating less calories because you are balanced and the body is in partnership with you. The truth is that it doesn't take a lot of calories to live at your desired weight. In today's hostile food environment, your desired weight is unattainable unless you equip yourself to know how to live balanced. Otherwise, small portions become about deprivation and self control.

This chapter is designed to give you a roadmap – hopefully to give you an awareness as to what it takes to live the life you deserve.

Here's How to Apply the Six Steps.

Step one
1. Analyze Your Current Foods.

The first step is to decide if the foods you are currently eating are helping or hurting you. What you will find is that most of us eat about 12 different foods, prepared and cooked in different ways. It takes a little brain power to break down some of your recipes into individual protein and fiber servings. List the foods you currently eat and calculate how close they meet the six steps.

Foods & Amount	Calories	Protein (g)	Fiber (g)

Step two
2. Calculate Your Portions For the Life You Want to live.

To be a certain weight, assuming it is reasonable, the big question is: can you live the lifestyle that is required at your desired weight? Anyone can lose weight on a food plan for a 100-pound person, but is this really the solution? Why are you trying to live a lie? Sure, weight-loss programs get the weight off quickly (but not permanently), and there is a cost to your metabolism and self worth when you try and live at a caloric value that is unrealistic. Why not teach yourself to live the weight you want to be instead of the weight you will never be?

Portion sizes matter, and the number of calories in those portions matter, the problem is a calorie-restrictive diet makes you feel deprived and miserable. The solution is to let the six steps work for you to keep you balanced. You eat smart portions, because you are empowered to know what a smart portion is. Smart portions mean fewer calories, naturally. Fewer calories eventually mean you weigh less not because you are on a diet, but because you know how to live the life of what you weigh being balanced.

If You Don't Follow the Six Steps, It Will Be Impossible to Maintain a Lean Life

I hate to sound negative, but there is too much going against you. Food addiction alone will make it very unlikely that you will succeed. Your environment is stacked against you. Corporations have too much to gain from your failure. You have to be smart about keeping balanced, and you have to be empowered to stay there.

Work the Numbers

For those who are impatient for the six step process to happen naturally, you can work the numbers of your desired weight and teach yourself to live that life. First, you have to calculate the number of calories needed to live the life you want. From there you can apply the six steps. When there is no food addiction or feelings of deprivation, it is very easy to live with the calories of your perfect weight.

1. Calculate Your Base Calories

Your body burns a certain number of calories for just staying alive. It is called **base calories.**

Base calories = Resting Rate

Resting rate is approximately 60%-75% of total daily calories burned. The higher percentage of muscle mass, the more calories you burn at rest. An increase in muscle tissue can increase resting calories by as much as 100-500 calories more per day.

Your desired weight _____ **+ add a zero =** _____

Calories needed to stay alive at your desired weight (metabolic rate=resting rate)

Example:

Desired weight = 150 pounds + 0 = 1,500 base calories

Calories needed to keep a 150 lb person alive. This is their resting rate.

2. Calculate Daily Activity Calories

Daily activity is approximately 25%-40% ot total daily calories burned.

Daily activity is based on how much physical movement the body does during the day. Your daily activity calories are added to your base calories to get the total calories for the day. This can be difficult to calculate and discouraging for those who stay very busy with multi tasks in their daily activity, that unfortunately, may not burn a lot of calories. The easiest way to figure out daily calories is based on how many <u>miles you walk in your daily routine</u>. This is not exercise, just the number of miles between your errands, work, and home. What makes it hard is that your metabolism can be higher or lower by as much as 300-400 calories.

If you are very muscular, then your metabolism can burn 300-400 more calories per day doing the same activity as someone who is fat. If you have poor eating habits and have trained your body to eat only once a day, this can also lower your metabolism, where you burn less calories per day. As I said, it is really hard to get an exact figure for the number of calories you burn for moving through your day, and it can change based on your lifestyle. The only sure thing is that the body burns calories when moving your flesh over a certain distance, and the easiest way to know this is to estimate the number of steps or miles you move your body during your daily routine.

For now, we are going to use a more consistent method that is much easier to measure, that estimates daily activity by the number of steps you move through out your normal routine. Keep in mind, exercise is considered extra and is added to the base and activity calories.

	Light Activity	Medium Activity	High Activity
Distance (miles)	Less than 1 mile	1-3	3-5
Distance (steps)	2,000	2,000-6,000	6,000-10,000
Multiple Rate	.2 – .3	.3 – .5	.5 – .7

Multiply

Base Calories X Multiple Rate = Calories Burned in Activity

Assume the same person in example #1. walks 2,000 steps per day. This person would burn approximately 450 calories that would be added to their base calories to figure the total amount of calories needed to live life in the six steps.

> Base Calories **(1,500)** X .Multiple Rate **(.3)** = Calories Burned in Activity **(450)**

Add calories burned in activity to your base rate to get your total daily calories burned.

1,500
+450
1,950 total calories to live the life of a 150 pound person.

If you lived the six steps at 1,950 calories, you would eventually weigh 150 pounds. The key is to live the life of what you want to be. The six steps are the only way that this will be possible because it is about living a lifestyle, not a diet.

3. Calculate Calories Burned with Exercise

One factor we know for sure is that there is a direct relationship between the number of heart beats and the number of calories burned during that period. Yes, as I said before, once you become more muscular and change your lifestyle, you will get a faster metabolism that burns fat more easily. But this is impossible to measure and I'd rather let that be an extra bonus. For our purposes, we need to give you a lifestyle that you can feel comfortable living and with consistent numbers. If you end up burning more fat than you expected, and have to add more food to your program, then good for you!

How many minutes at Target Heart Rate determine calories burned?

Calories Burned in Aerobic Exercise for 30 Minutes

Intensity	Light	Medium	Vigorous
Target Heart Rate	Less than 55%	65%–85%	More than 85%
Calories Burned	150-200	200-300	300-500

Exercising for longer continuous durations at target heart rate (60%-80%) encourages the body to be efficient at burning fat.

With Exercise:

Assume this person exercises at 70% target heart rate for 30 minutes

1,950
<u>+300</u> (calories burned at target heart rate for 30 minutes)
2,200 calories burned with 30 minutes of target heart rate exercise during exercise.

After computing the number of calories that are needed to live the life you want, at the weight you want, now you need to live the six steps in those calories.

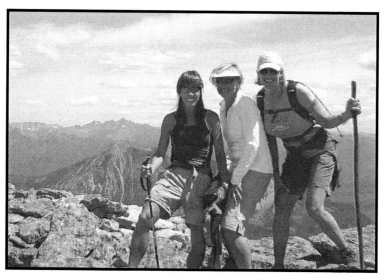

Myrna with friends mountain climbing 12,500 ft, Creste Butte Colorado.

Live the Six Steps

1. Water
Eight ounces per day

2. Protein/Fiber

No exercise
Current weight _____ x .4 _____ protein grams

Exercising 0-1 hours per day:
Current weight _____ x .5-.6 = _____ protein grams

Exercising 1-3 hours per day
Current weight _____ x .6-.8 = _____ protein grams

Exercising > 3 hours per day
Current weight _____ x .8-1.5 = _____ protein grams

Fiber
25-35+ grams per day

3. Essential Fats
Include Omega-3 fats in your day

4. Portions
200 Calorie Rule

5. Exercise
Healthy fit and/or Athletic fit

6. Empowerment
Power of association, behavior, affiliation and faith

This Book is Not Meant to Spoon-Feed You.

Anything spoon fed isn't real and it doesn't last.

You have to be empowered, educated and strong. That is the *truth* and that is the *way it is*.

This is a book about YOU and YOUR LIFE and what YOU ARE GOING TO DO to make it better!

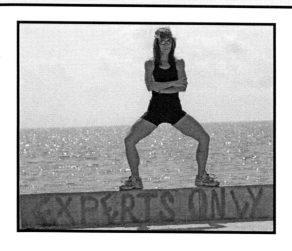

"Take Back Your Body!"